Ultimate Keto Air Fryer Diet Cookbook

Tasty and Delicious Seafood Meals to start Each Day

River Hunt

© Copyright 2020 - All rights reserved.

The content contained within this book may not be reproduced, duplicated or transmitted without direct written permission from the author or the publisher.

Under no circumstances will any blame or legal responsibility be held against the publisher, or author, for any damages, reparation, or monetary loss due to the information contained within this book. Either directly or indirectly.

Legal Notice:

This book is copyright protected. This book is only for personal use. You cannot amend, distribute, sell, use, quote or paraphrase any part, or the content within this book, without the consent of the author or publisher.

Disclaimer Notice:

Please note the information contained within this document is for educational and entertainment purposes only. All effort has been executed to present accurate, up to date, and reliable, complete information. No warranties of any kind are declared or implied. Readers acknowledge that the author is not engaging in the rendering of legal, financial, medical or professional advice. The content within this book has been derived from various sources. Please consult a licensed professional before attempting any techniques outlined in this book.

By reading this document, the reader agrees that under no circumstances is the author responsible for any losses, direct or indirect, which are incurred as a result of the use of information contained within this document, including, but not limited to, — errors, omissions, or inaccuracies.

Table of Contents

Golden Cod Fish Fillets 8

Tandoori Crispy Salmon 9

Smoked Salmon Taquitos 11

Lovely "Blackened" Catfish 13

Jamaican Catfish Fillets 15

Hot Sardine Cakes 17

Basil White Fish with Cheese 19

Herbed Crab Croquettes 21

Chinese Garlic Prawns 24

Cod Cornflakes Nuggets with Avocado Dip 26

Baked Trout en Papillote with Herbs 28

Ale-Battered Fish with Tartar Sauce 30

Peppery & Lemony Haddock 33

Oaty Fishcakes 34

Fiery Prawns 36

Buttered Crab Legs 38

Air-Fried Seafood 40

Cod Finger Pesto Sandwich 42

Hot Salmon Fillets with Broccoli 44

Crumbly Haddock Patties 46

Sesame Halibut Fillets 48

Delicious Coconut Shrimp 50

Asian Shrimp Medley 52

Breaded Scallops 54

Kimchi-Spiced Salmon 56

Mediterranean Salmon 58

Air Fried Tuna Sandwich 60

Greek-Style Fried Mussels 62

Greek-Style Salmon with Dill Sauce 64

Simple Creole Trout 66
Colorful Salmon and Fennel Salad 68
Fish Sticks with Vidalia Onions 70
Fish Cakes with Bell Pepper 72
Cajun Fish Cakes with Cheese 75
Monkfish with Sautéed Vegetables and Olives 76
Crispy Mustardy Fish Fingers 79
Roasted Mediterranean Snapper Fillets 81
Quick Thai Coconut Fish 83
Parmesan Chip-Crusted Tilapia 86
Classic Crab Cakes 87
Baked Sardines with Tangy Dipping Sauce 89
Classic Old Bay Fish with Cherry Tomatoes 91
Mom's Lobster Tails 93
Tuna Steak with Roasted Cherry Tomatoes 95
Vermouth and Garlic Shrimp Skewers 97
Cod and Shallot Frittata 99
Authentic Mediterranean Calamari Salad 101
Swordfish with Roasted Peppers and Garlic Sauce 104
Shrimp Kabobs with Cherry Tomatoes 105
Keto Cod Fillets 107

Golden Cod Fish Fillets

Cook Time:

20 minutes

Servings: 4

Iingredients:

4 cod fillets
2 tbsp olive oil
2 eggs, beaten
1 cup breadcrumbs
A pinch of salt
1 cup flour

Directions:

1. Preheat air fryer to 390 F. Mix breadcrumbs, olive oil, and salt in a bowl. In another bowl, place the eggs. Put the flour into a third bowl.

2. Toss the cod fillets in the flour, then in the eggs, and then in the breadcrumb mixture. Place them in the greased frying basket and Air Fryer for 9 minutes.

3. At the 5-minute mark, quickly turn the fillets. Once done, remove to a plate and serve with cilantro-yogurt sauce.

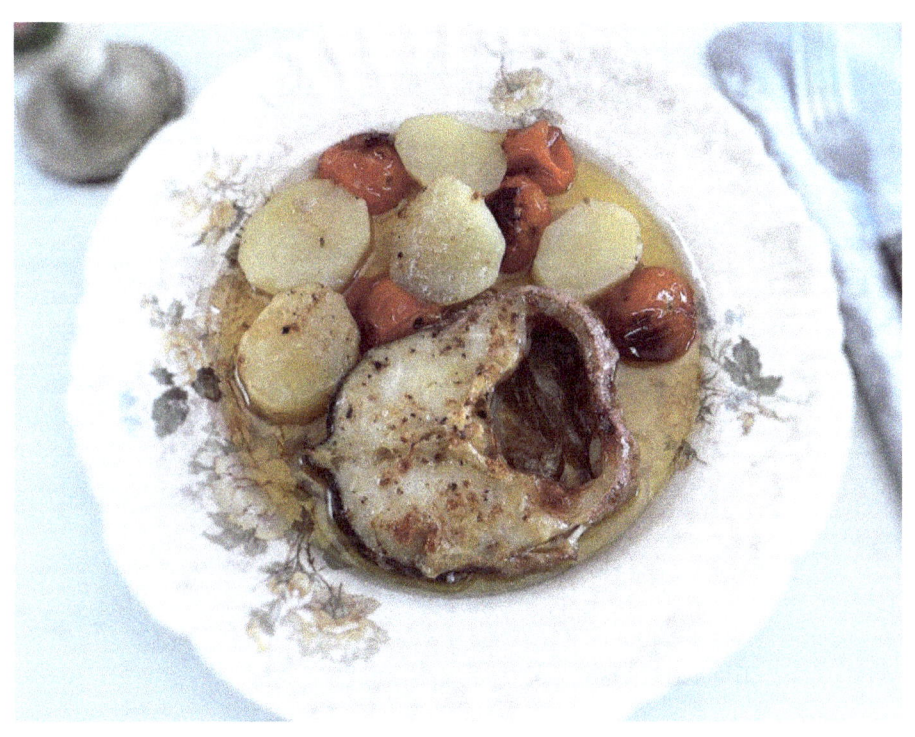

Tandoori Crispy Salmon

Cooking Time:
15 minutes
Servings: 3
Ingredients:

2 salmon fillets

1 tsp ginger powder

1 garlic clove, minced

½ green bell pepper, sliced

1 tsp sweet paprika, minced

1 tsp honey

1 tsp garam masala

1 tbsp fresh cilantro, chopped

¼ cup yogurt Juice and zest from

1 lime

DIirections:

1. In a bowl, mix all the ingredients, except for salmon and yogurt.

2. Season to taste and stir in the yogurt. Top the fillets with the mixture and let sit for 15 minutes.

3. Preheat air fryer to 400 F. Place the fillets into the greased frying basket and Bake for 12-15 minutes until nice and crispy. Serve on a bed of rice.

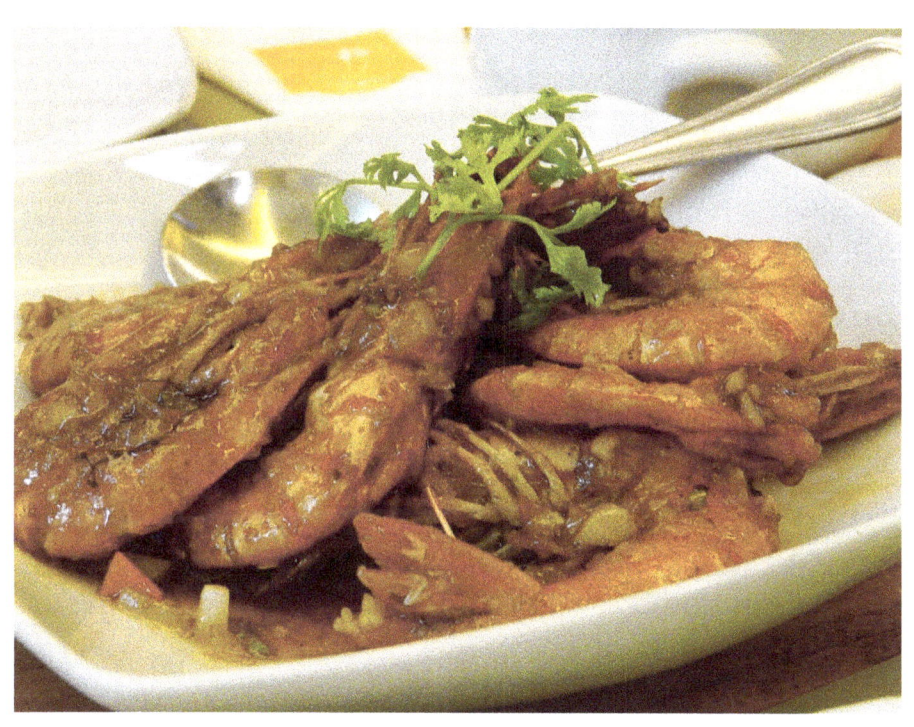

Smoked Salmon Taquitos

Cooking Time:

15 minutes

Servings: 4

Ingredients:

2 tbsp olive oil

1 lb smoked salmon, chopped

Salt to taste

1 tbsp taco seasoning

1 cup cheddar cheese, shredded

1 lime, juiced

½ cup fresh cilantro, chopped

8 corn tortillas

Directions:

1. Preheat air fryer to 390 F. In a bowl, mix salmon, taco seasoning, lime juice, cheddar cheese, salt, and cilantro.

2. Divide the mixture between the tortillas. Wrap the tortillas around the filling and place them in the greased air fryer basket.

3. Bake for 10 minutes, turning once halfway through. Serve with hot salsa.

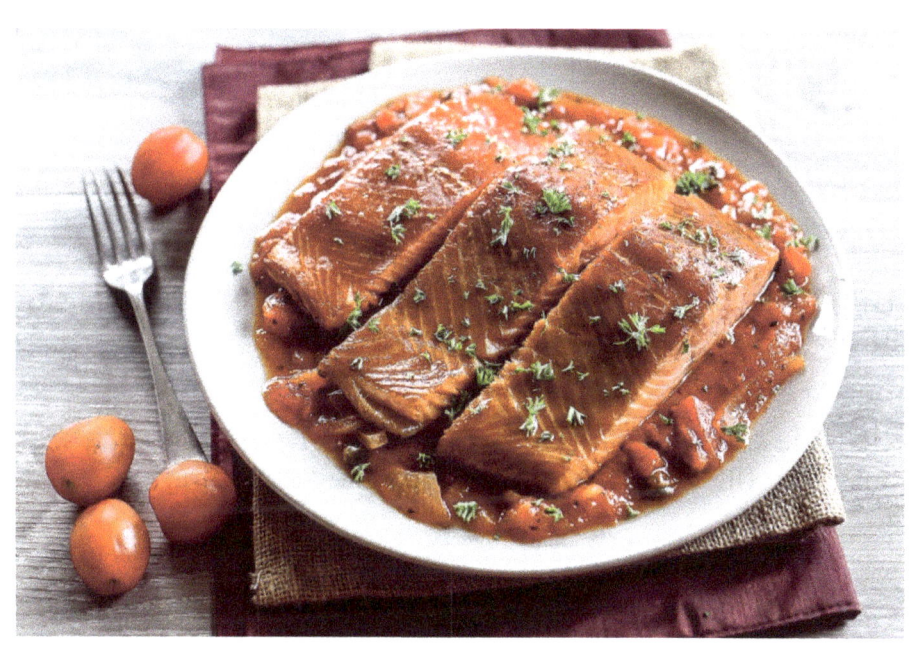

Lovely "Blackened" Catfish

Cooking Time:

15 minutes

Servings: 4

Ingredients:

2 catfish fillets

2 tsp blackening seasoning

Juice of 1 lime

2 tbsp butter, melted

1 garlic clove, minced

2 tbsp fresh cilantro, chopped

Directions:

1. Preheat air fryer to 360 F. In a bowl, mix garlic, lime juice, cilantro, and butter.

2. Divide the sauce into two parts, rub 1 part of the sauce onto fish fillets and sprinkle with the seasoning.

3. Place the fillets in the greased frying basket and Bake for 15 minutes, flipping once. Serve with the remaining sauce.

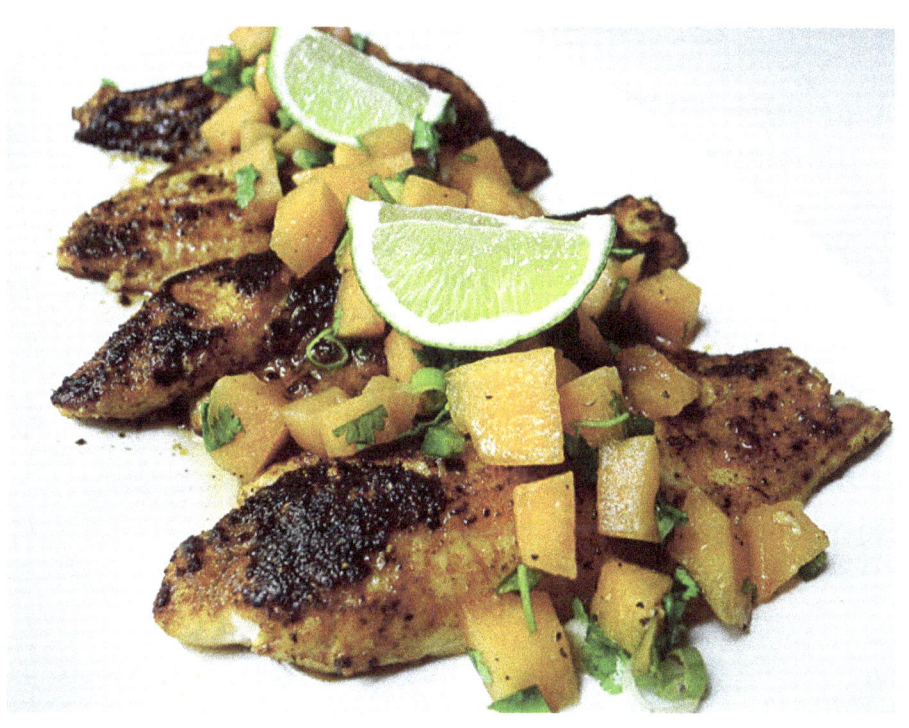

Jamaican Catfish Fillets

Cooking Time:

20 minutes

Servings: 4

Ingredients:

4 catfish fillets

2 tbsp olive oil

1 tsp paprika

1 tsp garlic powder

1 tsp dried basil

1 tbsp ground Jamaican allspice

½ lemon, juiced

Directions:

1. Preheat air fryer to 390 F. Spray the frying basket with cooking spray.

2. In a bowl, mix paprika, garlic powder, and Jamaican allspice seasoning. Rub the catfish fillets with the spice mixture.

3. Transfer to the frying basket and drizzle the olive oil. Air Fryer for 8 minutes, slide the basket out and turn the fillets. Cook further for 5 minutes until crispy. Sprinkle with lemon juice to serve.

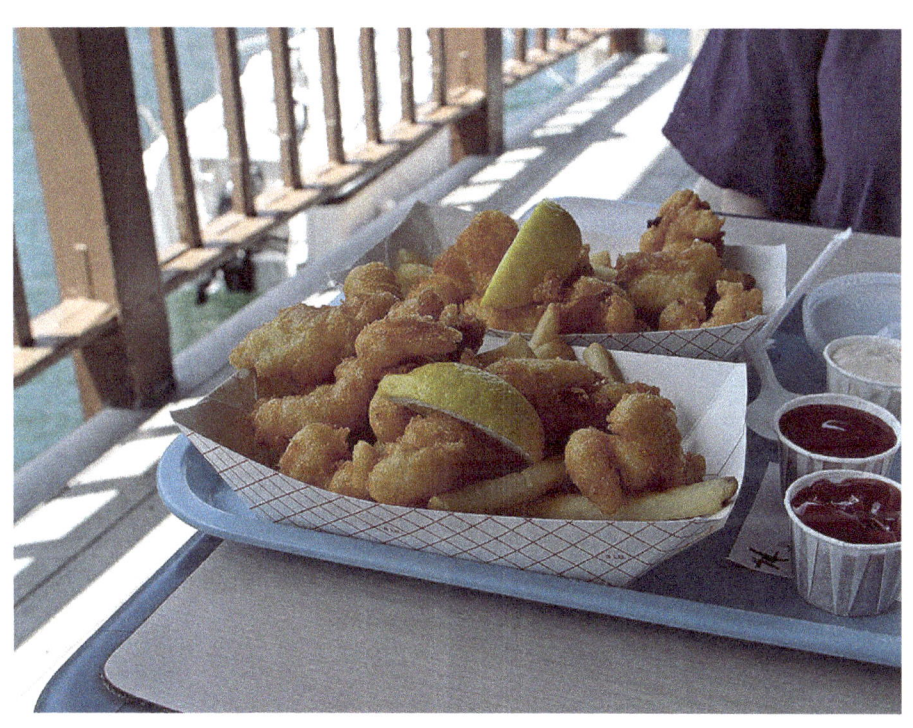

Hot Sardine Cakes

Cooking Time:
20 minutes

Servings: 4

Ingredients:

2 4-oz tins sardines, chopped

2 eggs, beaten

½ cup breadcrumbs

⅓ cup green onions, finely chopped

2 tbsp fresh parsley, chopped

1 tbsp mayonnaise

1 tsp sweet chili sauce

½ tsp paprika

Salt and black pepper to taste

2 tbsp olive oil

Directions:

1. In a bowl, add sardines, eggs, breadcrumbs, green onions, parsley, mayonnaise, chili sauce, paprika, salt, and black pepper.

2. Mix well with hands. Shape into 8 cakes and brush them lightly with olive oil.

3. Air Fryer in the fryer for 8 minutes at 390 F, shaking once halfway through cooking. Serve warm.

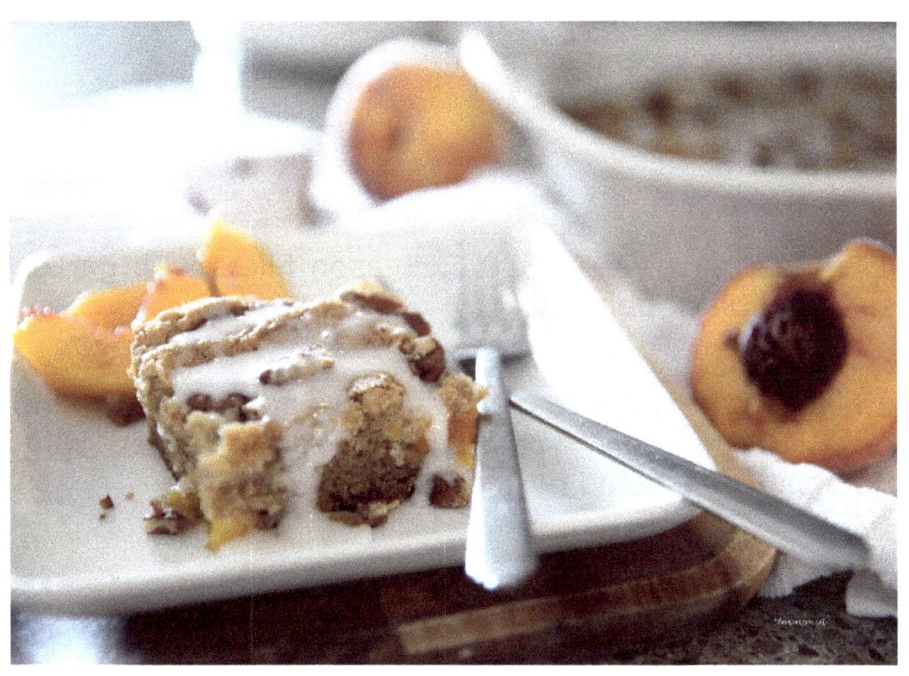

Basil White Fish with Cheese

Cooking Time:

15 minutes:

Servings:4

Ingredients:

2 tbsp fresh basil, chopped

1 tsp garlic powder

2 tbsp Romano cheese, grated

Salt and black pepper to taste

4 white fish fillets

Direction:

1. Preheat air fryer to 350 F. Season fillets with garlic, salt, and black pepper.

2. Place in the greased frying basket and Air Fryer them for 8-10 minutes, flipping once. Serve topped with Romano cheese and basil.

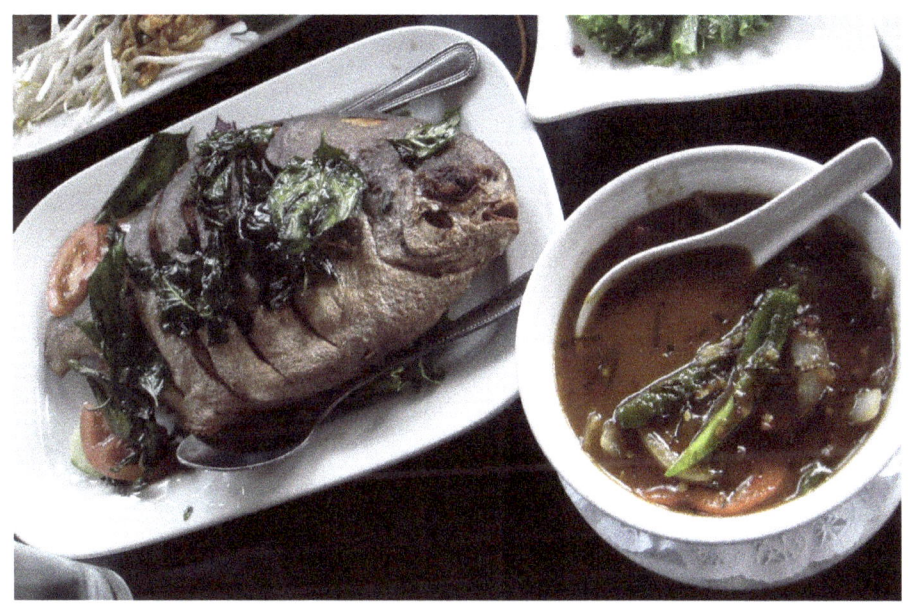

Herbed Crab Croquettes

Cooking Time:
25 minutes
Servings: 4
Ingredients:
1 ½ lb lump crab meat
⅓ cup sour cream
⅓ cup mayonnaise
1 red pepper, finely chopped
⅓ cup red onion, chopped
½ celery stalk, chopped
1 tsp fresh tarragon, chopped
1 tsp fresh chives, chopped
1 tsp fresh parsley, chopped
1 tsp cayenne pepper
1 ½ cups breadcrumbs
2 tsp olive oil
1 cup flour
3 eggs, beaten
Salt to taste Lemon wedges to serve

Directions:

1. Heat olive oil in a skillet over medium heat and sauté red pepper, onion, and celery for 5 minutes or until sweaty and translucent.

2. Turn off the heat. Pour the breadcrumbs and salt on a plate.

3.In 2 separate bowls, add the flour and beaten eggs, respectively, set aside. In a separate bowl, add crabmeat, mayo, sour cream, tarragon, chives, parsley, cayenne pepper, and vegetable sauteed mix.

4. Form bite-sized oval balls from the mixture and place them onto a plate. Preheat air fryer to 390 F. Dip each crab meatball in the beaten eggs and press them in the breadcrumb mixture.

5.Place the croquettes in the greased fryer basket without overcrowding. Cook for 10 minutes until golden brown, shaking once halfway through. Serve hot with lemon wedges.

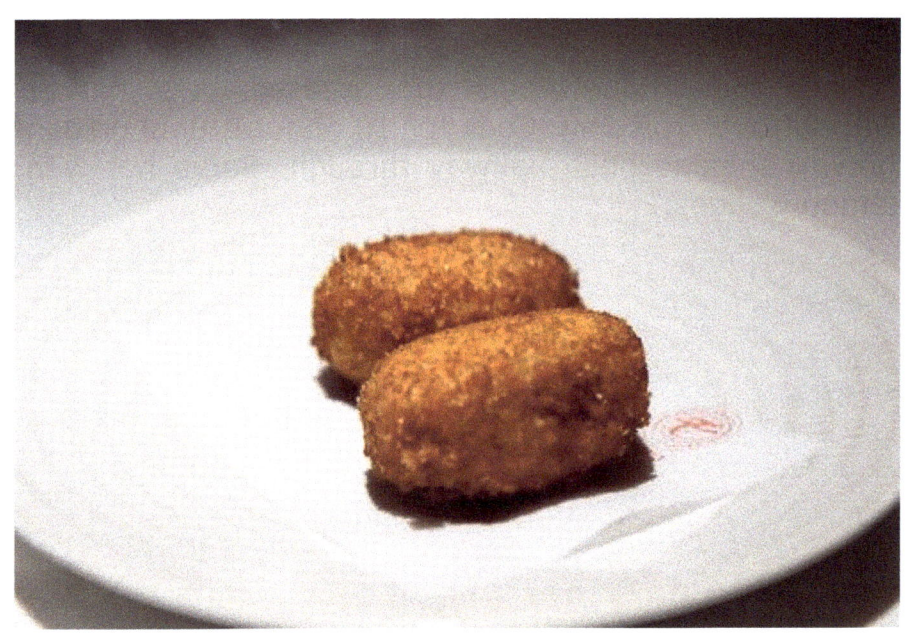

Chinese Garlic Prawns

Cook Time:

20minutes

Servings:**4**

Ingredients:

1 lb prawns, peeled and deveined
Juice of 1 lemon
1 tsp sugar
2 tbsp peanut oil
2 tbsp cornstarch
2 scallions, chopped
¼ tsp Chinese powder
1 red chili pepper, minced
Salt and black pepper to taste
4 garlic cloves, minced

Directions:

1.In a Ziploc bag, mix lemon juice, sugar, black pepper, 1 tbsp peanut oil, cornstarch, Chinese powder, and salt. Add in prawns and massage gently to coat.

2.Let sit for 20 minutes. Heat the remaining peanut oil in a pan over medium heat and sauté garlic, scallions, and red chili pepper for 5 minutes.

3.Preheat air fryer to 390 F. Place the marinated prawns in a baking dish and cover with the sautéed vegetables. Air Fryer for 10 minutes, shaking once halfway through, until nice and crispy. Serve warm.

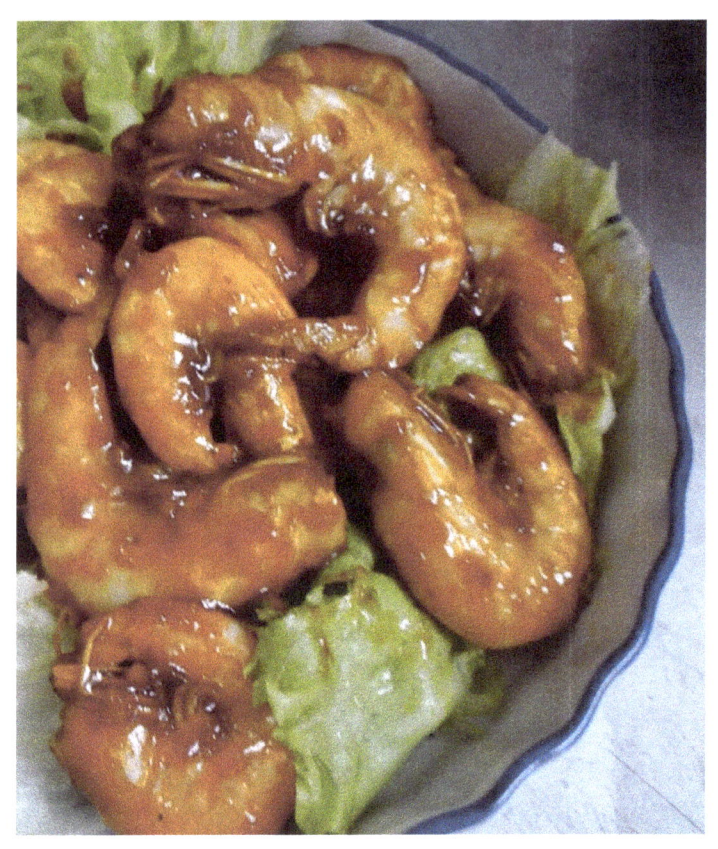

Cod Cornflakes Nuggets with Avocado Dip

Cooking Time:
20 minutes
Servings: 4
Ingredients:
1¼ lb cod fillets, cut into 4 chunks each
½ cup flour
2 eggs, beaten
1 cup cornflakes
1 tbsp olive oil
Salt and black pepper to taste
1 avocado, chopped
1 lime, juiced

Directions:

1. Mash the avocado with a fork in a small bowl. Stir in lime juice and salt and set aside. Place olive oil and cornflakes in a food processor and process until crumbed.

2. Season the fish with salt and pepper. Preheat air fryer to 350 F. Place flour, eggs and cornflakes in separate dishes.

3. Toss the fish with flour, dip in eggs, then coat well with cornflakes. Air Fryer for 15 minutes until golden. Serve with avocado dip.

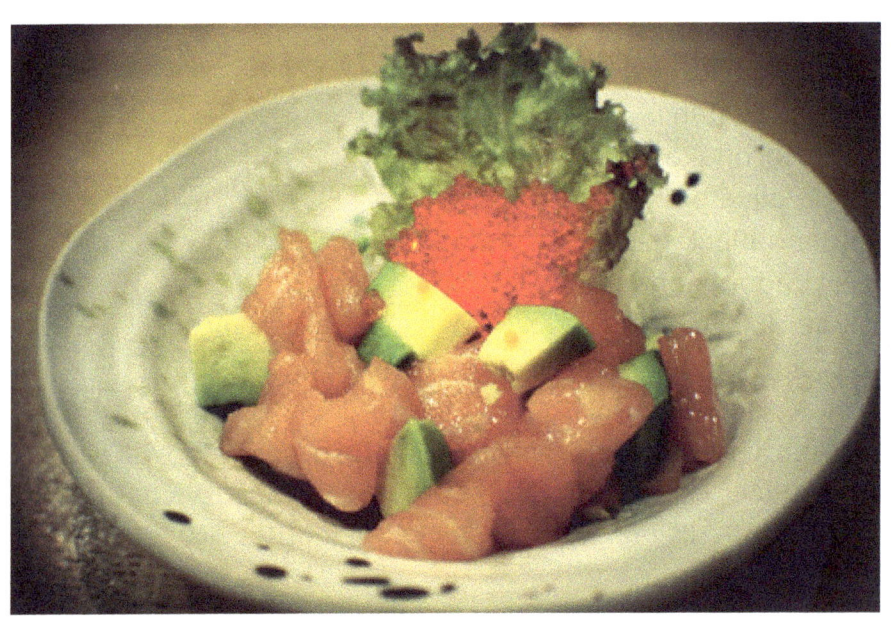

Baked Trout en Papillote with Herbs

Cooking Time:

20 minutes

Servings: 4

Ingredients:

1 whole trout, scaled and cleaned

¼ bulb fennel, sliced

½ brown onion, sliced

1 tbsp fresh parsley, chopped

1 tbsp fresh dill, chopped

1 tbsp olive oil

1 lemon, sliced

Salt and black pepper to taste

Directions:

1. In a bowl, add the onion, parsley, dill, fennel, and garlic. Mix and drizzle with olive oil. Preheat air fryer to 350 F.

2. Open the cavity of the fish and fill with the fennel mixture.

3. Wrap the fish completely in parchment paper and then in foil. Place the fish in the frying basket and Bake for 14 minutes.

4. Remove the paper and foil and top with lemon slices to serve

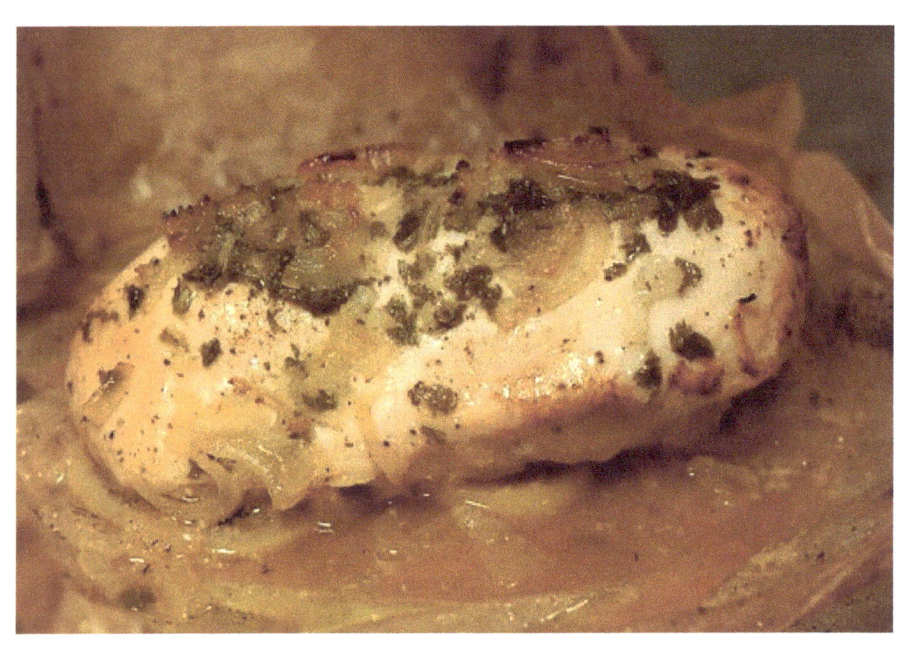

Ale-Battered Fish with Tartar Sauce

Cooking Time:
20 minutes

Servings: 4

Ingredients:

4 lemon wedges
2 eggs
1 cup ale beer
1 cup flour
Salt and black pepper to taste
4 white fish fillets
½ cup light mayonnaise
½ cup Greek yogurt
2 dill pickles, chopped
1 tbsp capers
1 tbsp fresh dill, roughly chopped
Lemon wedges to serve

Directions:

1. Preheat air fryer to 390 F. Beat the eggs in a bowl along with ale beer, salt, and black pepper. Pat dry the fish fillets with paper towels and dredge them in the flour.

2. Shake off the excess flour. Dip in the egg mixture and then in the flour again. Spray with cooking spray and add to the frying basket.

3. Air Fryer for 10 minutes, flipping once. In a bowl, mix mayonnaise, yogurt, capers, salt, and dill pickles. Serve the fish with the sauce and freshly cut lemon wedges.

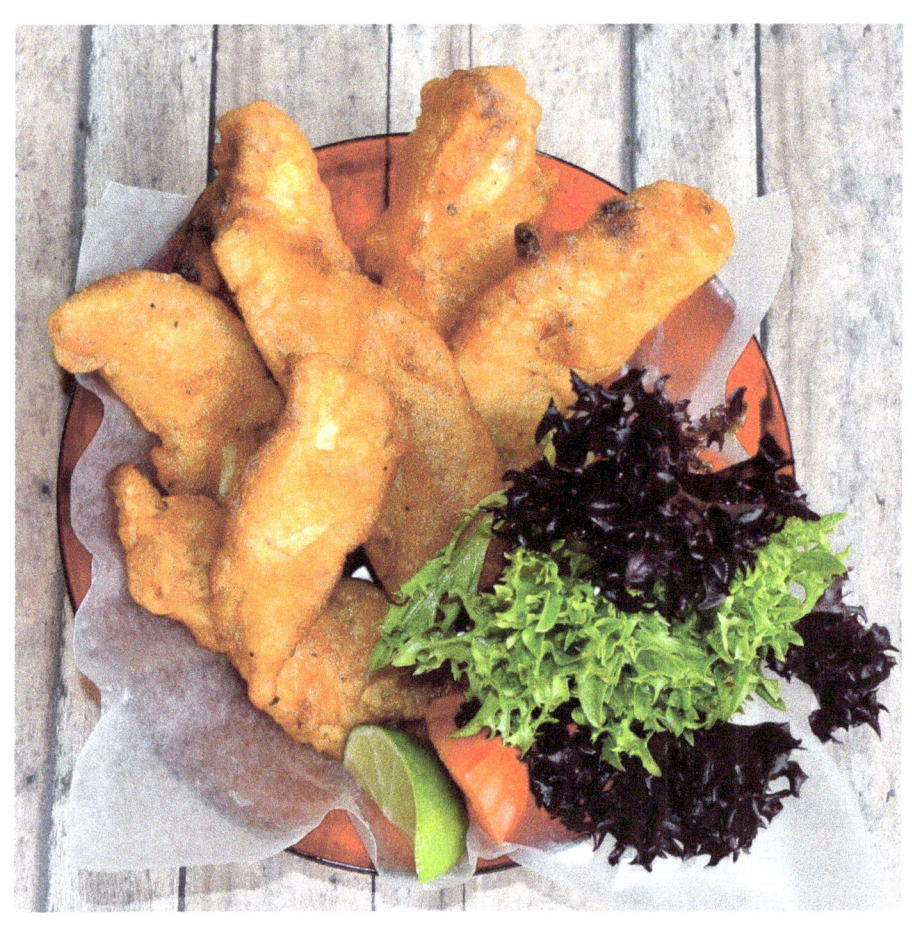

Peppery & Lemony Haddock

Cooking Time:
20 minutes
Servings: 4
Ingredients:
4 haddock fillets
1 cup breadcrumbs
2 tbsp lemon juice
Salt and black pepper to taste
¼ cup potato flakes
2 eggs, beaten
¼ cup Parmesan cheese, grated
3 tbsp flour

Directions:

1. In a bowl, combine flour, salt, and pepper. In another bowl, combine breadcrumbs, Parmesan cheese, and potato flakes.

2. Dip fillets in the flour first, then in the eggs, and coat them with the cheese crumbs. Place in the frying basket and Air Fryer for 14-16 minutes at 370 F, flipping once. Serve with lemon juice.

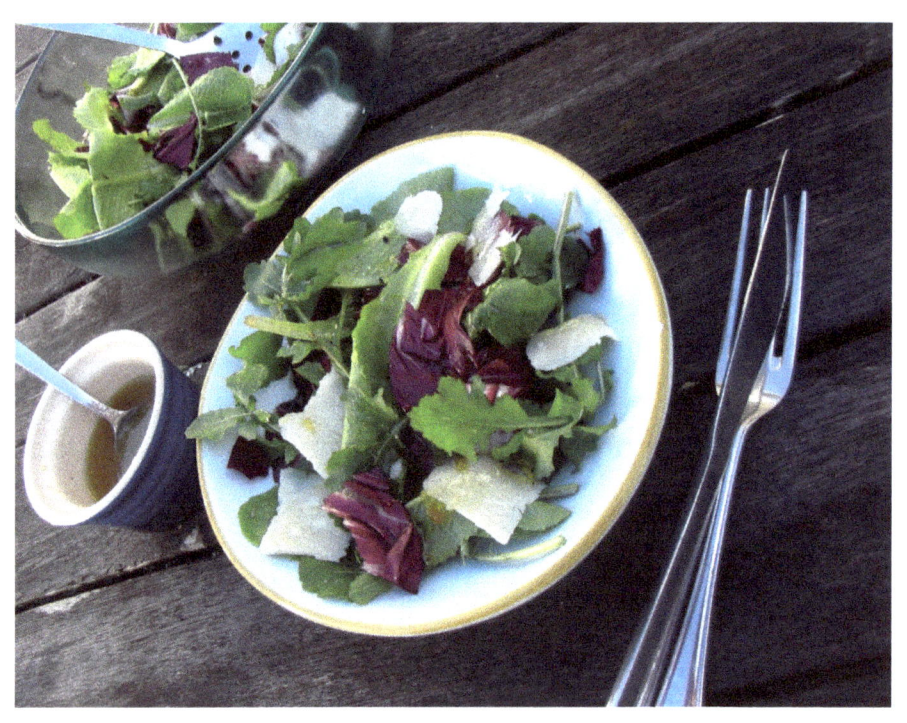

Oaty Fishcakes

Cooking Time:

20 minutes

Servings: 4

Ingredients:

4 potatoes, cooked and mashed

2 salmon fillets, cubed

1 haddock fillet, cubed

1 tsp Dijon mustard

½ cup oats

2 tbsp fresh dill, chopped

2 tbsp olive oil

Salt and black pepper to taste

Directions:

1. Preheat air fryer to 400 F. Boil salmon and haddock cubes in a pot filled with salted water over medium heat for 5 minutes.

2. Drain, cool, and pat dry. Flake or shred and add to a bowl.

3. Mix in mashed potatoes, mustard, oats, dill, salt, and pepper.

4. Shape into balls and flatten to make patties. Brush with olive oil and arrange them on the bottom of the frying basket.

5. Bake for 10 minutes, flipping once halfway through. Let cool before serving.

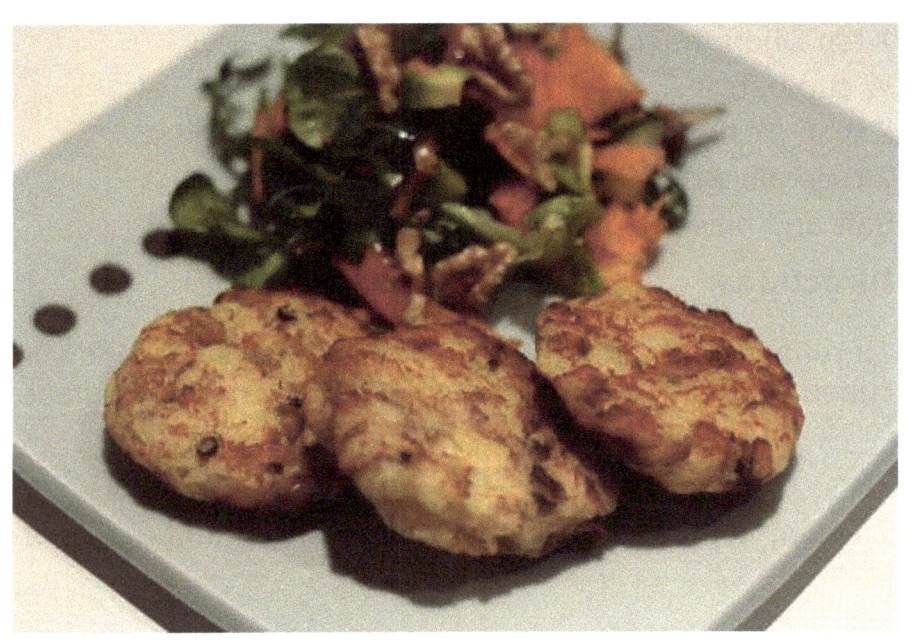

Fiery Prawns

Cooking Time:
20 minutes

Servings:4

Ingredients:

8 prawns, cleaned

Salt and black pepper to taste

½ tsp ground cayenne pepper

½ tsp red chili flakes

½ tsp ground cumin

½ tsp garlic powder

Directions:

1. In a bowl, season the prawns with salt and black pepper.

2. Sprinkle with cayenne pepper, chili flakes, cumin, and garlic, and stir to coat.

3. Spray the frying basket with oil and lay the prawns in an even layer.

4. Air Fryer for 8 minutes at 340 F, turning once halfway through. Serve with fresh sweet chili sauce.

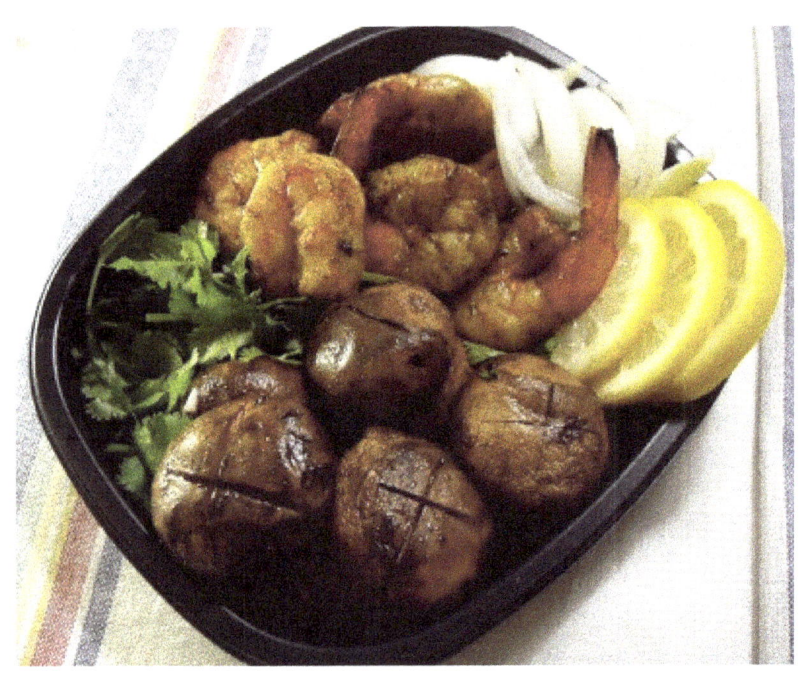

Buttered Crab Legs

Cooking Time:
20 minutes
Servings: 4
Ingredients:
3 lb crab legs
2 tbsp butter, melted
1 tbsp fresh parsley

Directions:

1. Preheat air fryer to 380 F. Place the crab legs in the greased air fryer basket and Air Fryer for 10 minutes, shaking once.

2. Pour the butter over crab legs, sprinkle with parsley, and serve.

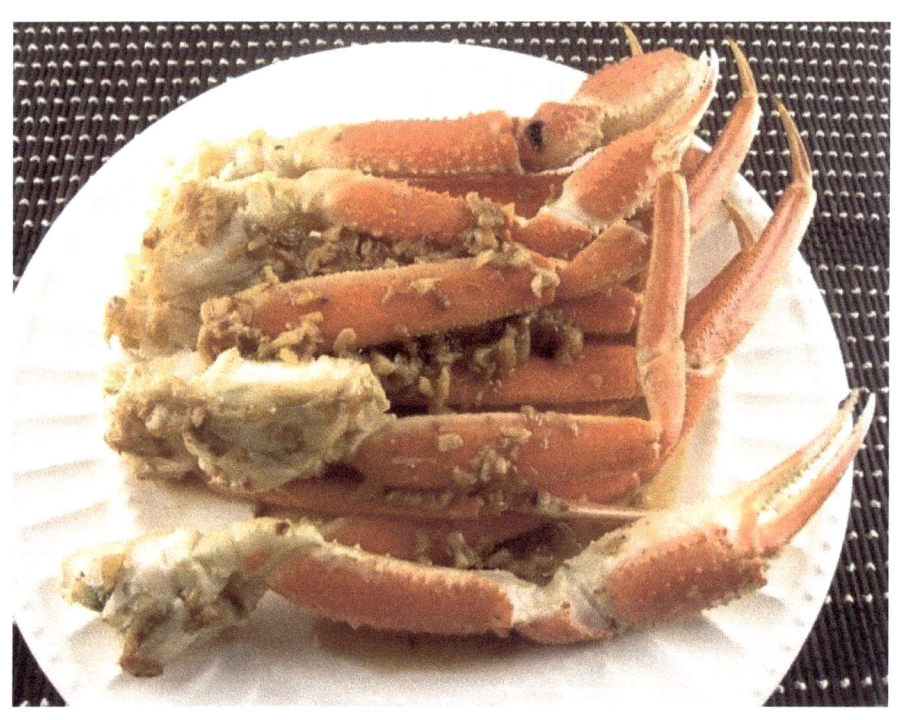

Air-Fried Seafood

Cook Time:

15 minutes

Servings: 4

Ingredients:

1 lb fresh scallops, mussels, fish fillets, prawns, shrimp

2 eggs

Salt and black pepper to taste

1 cup breadcrumbs mixed with the zest of 1 lemon

Directions:

1. Beat the eggs with salt and pepper in a bowl. Dip in each piece of seafood and then coat with breadcrumbs.

2. Place in the greased air fryer basket and Air Fryer for 10-12 minutes at 400 F, turning once.

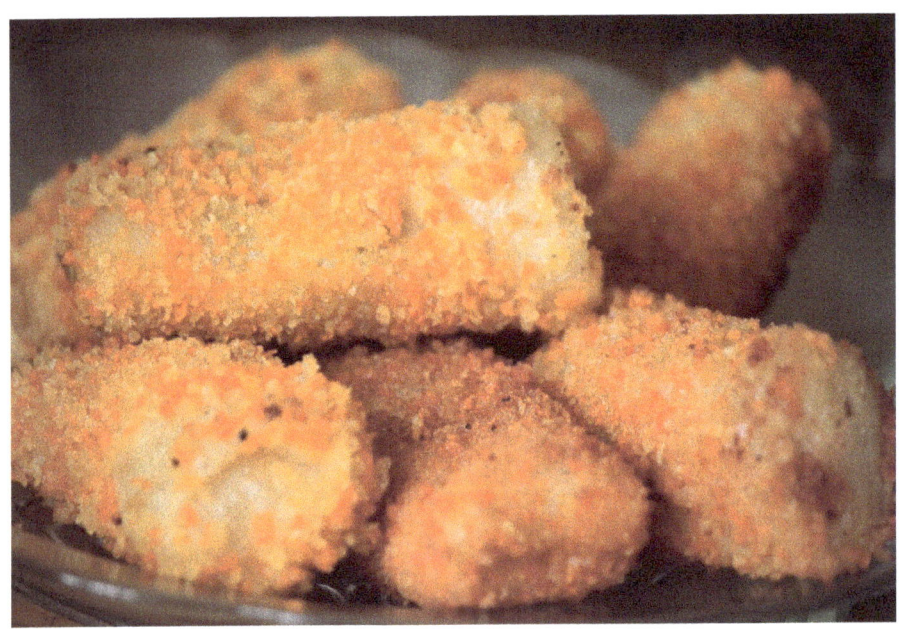

Cod Finger Pesto Sandwich

Cooking Time:

20 minutes

Servings: 4

Ingredients:

4 cod fillets

4 bread rolls

1 cup breadcrumbs

4tbsp pesto sauce

4 lettuce leaves

Salt and black pepper to taste

Directions:

1. Preheat air fryer to 370 F. Season the fillets with salt and black pepper and coat them with breadcrumbs.

2. Arrange them into the greased air fryer basket and Bake for 12-15 minutes, flipping once.

3. Cut the bread rolls in half. Divide lettuce leaves between the bottom halves and place the fillets over. Spread pesto sauce on top of the fillets and cover with the remaining halves to serve.

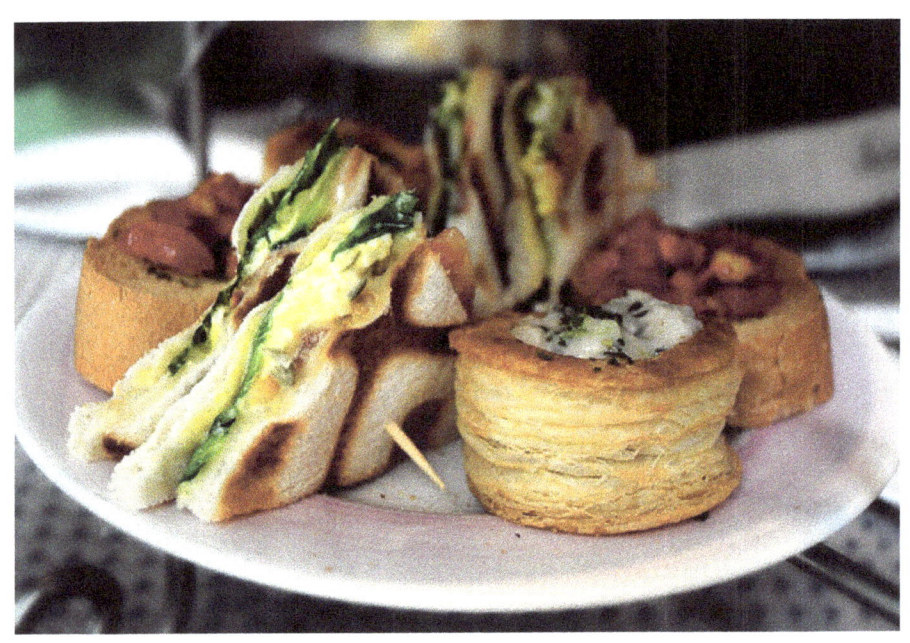

Hot Salmon Fillets with Broccoli

Cooking Time:

25minutes

Servings: 4

Ingredients:

2 salmon fillets

2 tsp olive oil

Juice of 1 lime

1 tsp chili flakes

Salt and black pepper to taste

5 oz broccoli florets, steamed

1 tbsp soy sauce

Directions:

1. In a bowl, add half of the olive oil, lime juice, chili flakes, salt, and black pepper; rub the mixture onto fillets.

2. Lay the florets into your air fryer and drizzle with the remaining olive oil.

3. Arrange the fillets on top and Bake at 340 F for 14 minutes, flipping once. Drizzle the florets with soy sauce and serve with fish.

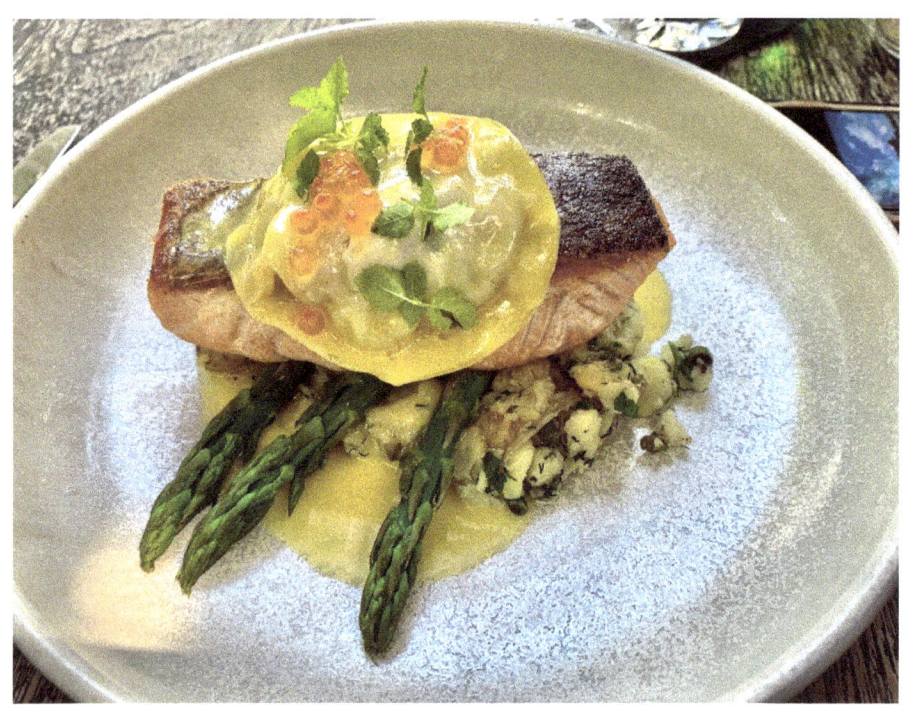

Crumbly Haddock Patties
Cook Time:
15minutes
Servings:2
INGREDIENTS

8 oz haddock, cooked and flaked
2 potatoes, cooked and mashed
2 tbsp green olives, pitted and chopped
1 tbsp fresh cilantro, chopped
1 tsp lemon zest
1 egg, beaten

Directions:

1.Mix haddock, zest, olives, cilantro, egg, and potatoes. Shape into patties and chill for 60 minutes.

2.Preheat air fryer to 350 F. Place the patties in the greased baking basket and Air Fryer for 12-14 minutes, flipping once halfway through cooking. Serve with green salad.

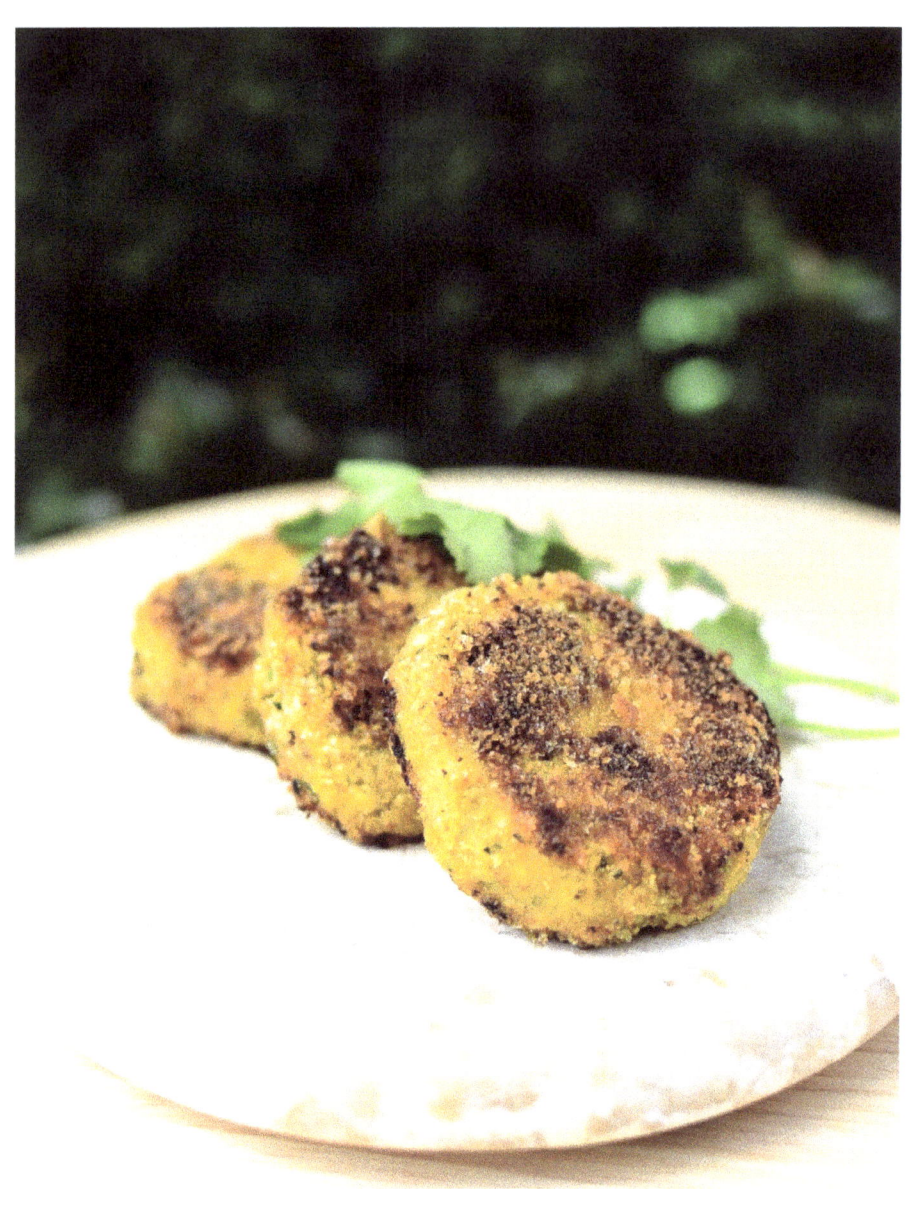

Sesame Halibut Fillets

Cooking Time:
20minutes
Servings:4
Ingredients:
4 halibut fillets
4 biscuits, crumbled
3 tbsp flour
1 egg, beaten
Salt and black pepper to taste
¼ tsp dried rosemary
3 tbsp olive oil
2 tbsp sesame seeds

Directions:

1. Preheat air fryer to 390 F. In a bowl, combine flour, black pepper, and salt.

2. In another bowl, combine sesame seeds, crumbled biscuits, olive oil, and rosemary.

3. Dip the fish fillets into the flour mixture first, then into the beaten egg. Finally, coat them with the sesame mixture.

4. Arrange on the greased frying basket and Air Fryer for 8 minutes. Flip the fillets and cook for 4-5 more minutes. Serve immediately.

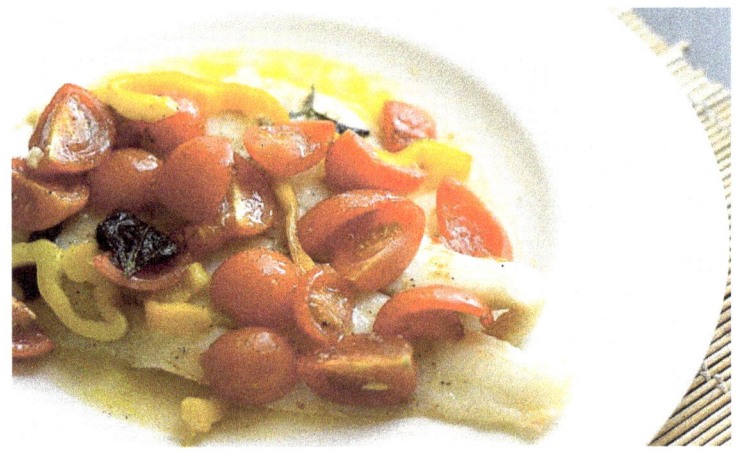

Delicious Coconut Shrimp

Cooking Time:

30 minutes

Servings: 4

Ingredients:

8 large shrimp, peeled and deveined

½ cup breadcrumbs

8 oz coconut milk

½ cup coconut, shredded

Salt to taste ½ cup orange jam

1 tsp mustard

1 tbsp honey

½ tsp cayenne pepper

¼ tsp hot sauce

Directions:

1. Combine breadcrumbs, cayenne pepper, shredded coconut, and salt in a bowl. Dip the shrimp in the coconut milk, and then in the coconut crumbs.

2. Arrange on a lined sheet and Bake in the air fryer for 12 minutes at 350 F. Whisk jam, honey, hot sauce, and mustard in a bowl. Serve with the shrimp.

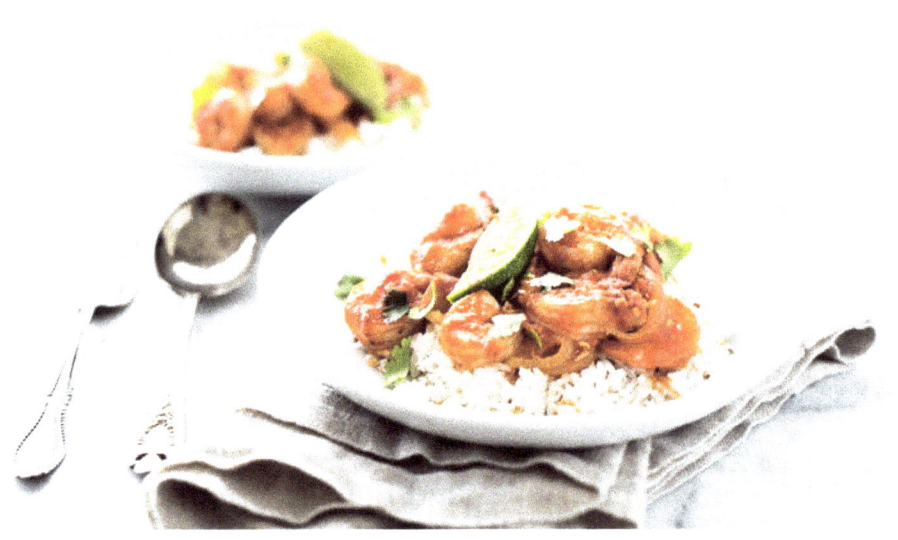

Asian Shrimp Medley

Cook Time:

20 minutes

Servings: 4

Ingredients:

1 lb shrimp, peeled and deveined
2 whole onions, chopped
3 tbsp butter
1 tbsp sugar
2 tbsp soy sauce
2 cloves garlic, chopped
2 tsp lime juice
1 tsp ginger paste

Directions:

1. Melt butter in a frying pan over medium heat and stir-fry the onions for 3 minutes until translucent.

2. Mix in the lime juice, soy sauce, ginger paste, garlic, and sugar and stir for 1-2 minutes. Let cool and then pour the mixture over the shrimp.

3. Cover and let marinate for 30 minutes in the fridge. Preheat air fryer to 380 F.

4. Transfer the shrimp with marinade to a baking dish and Air Fryer in the fryer for 12 minutes, shaking once halfway through. Serve warm.

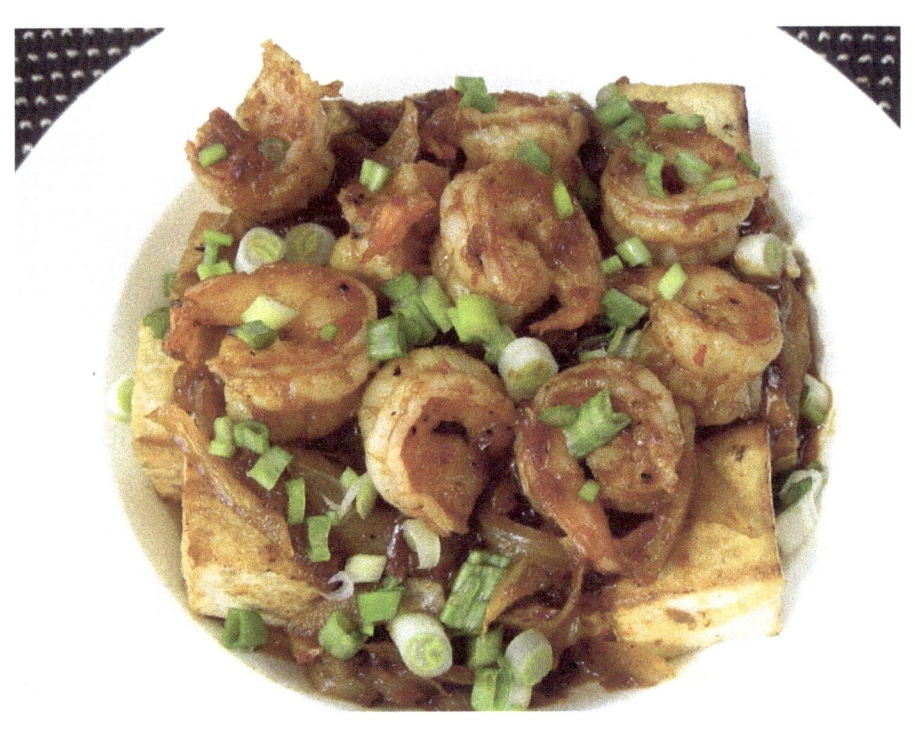

Breaded Scallops

Cooking Time:
15 minutes
Servings: 2
Ingredients:
1lb fresh scallops
3 tbsp flour
Salt and black pepper to taste
1 egg, lightly beaten
1 cup breadcrumbs
2 tbsp olive oil
½ tsp fresh parsley, chopped

Directions:

1. Coat the scallops with flour. Dip into the egg, then into the breadcrumbs.

2. Brush with olive oil and place into the frying basket. Air Fryer for 6-8 minutes at 360 F, shaking once. Serve topped with parsley. Enjoy!

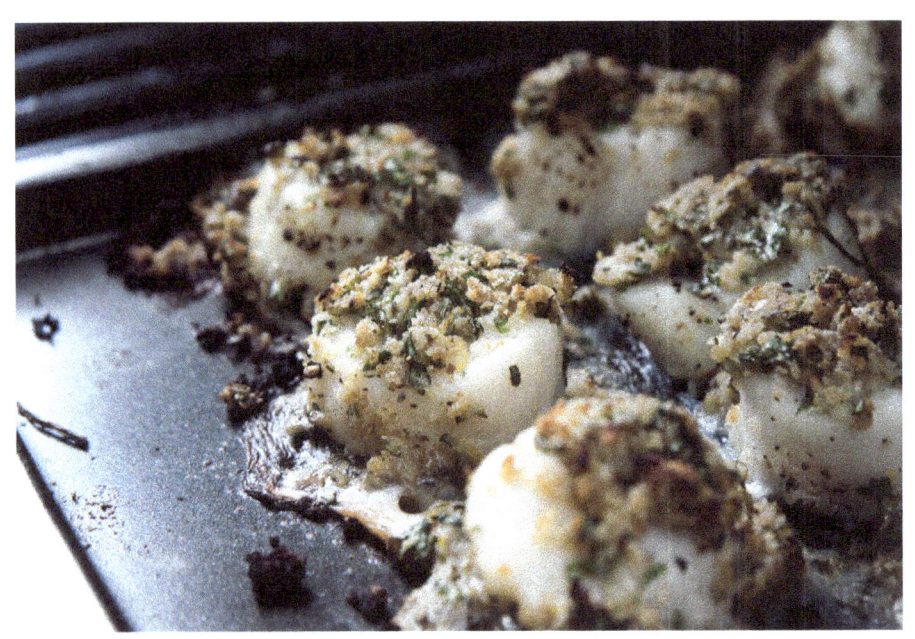

Kimchi-Spiced Salmon

Cooking Time:

15 minutes

Servings: 4

Ingredients:

1 tbsp soy sauce

2 tbsp sesame oil

2 tbsp mirin

1 tbsp ginger puree

1 tsp kimchi spice

1 tsp sriracha sauce

2 lb salmon fillets

1 lime, cut into wedges

Directions:

1. Preheat air fryer to 350 F. Grease the air fryer basket with cooking spray.

2. In a bowl, mix together soy sauce, mirin, ginger puree, kimchi spice, and sriracha sauce. Add the salmon fillets and toss to coat.

3. Place in the air fryer basket and drizzle with sesame oil. Air Fryer for 10 minutes, flipping once halfway through. Garnish with lime wedges and serve

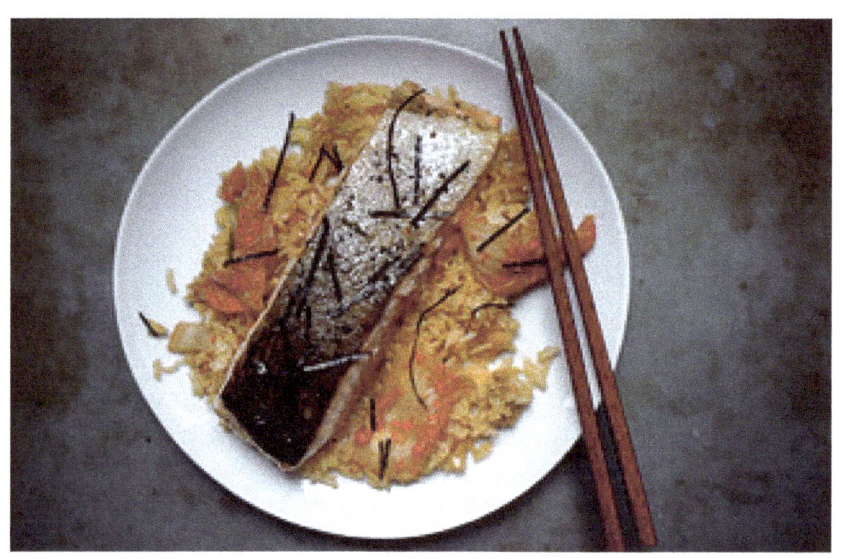

Mediterranean Salmon

Cook Time:

15 minutes

Servings: 2

Ingredients:

2 salmon fillets

Salt and black pepper to taste

1 lemon, cut into wedges

8 asparagus spears, trimmed

Directions:

1. Rinse and pat dry the fillets with a paper towel. Coat the fish generously on both sides with cooking spray.

2. Season fish and asparagus with salt and pepper. Arrange fish in the frying basket and lay the asparagus around the fish.

3. AirFry for 10-12 minutes at 350 F, flipping once. Serve with lemon wedges.

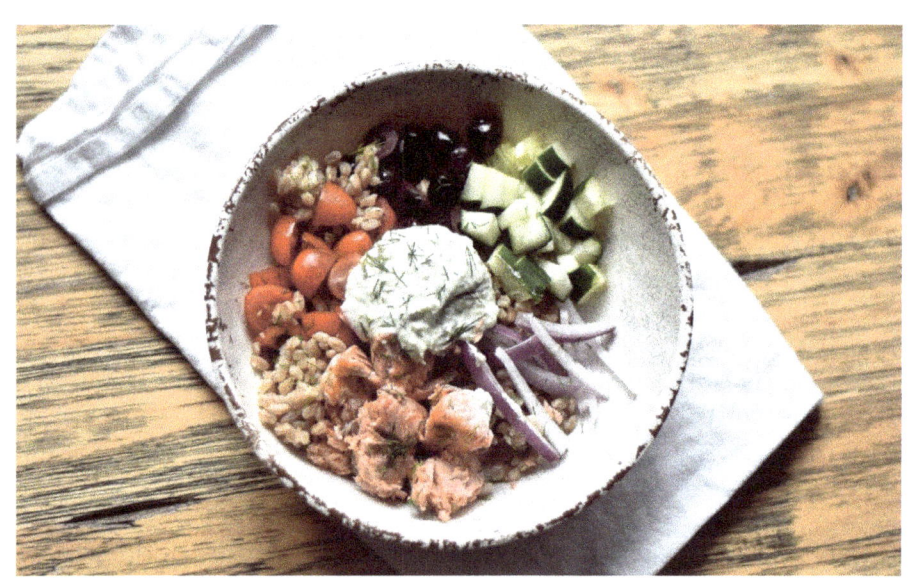

Air Fried Tuna Sandwich

Cooking Time:

15 minutes

Servings: 2

Ingredients:

4 white bread slices

1 5-oz can tuna, drained

½ onion, finely chopped

2 tbsp mayonnaise

1 cup mozzarella cheese, shredded

1 tbsp olive oil

Directions:

1. In a small bowl, mix tuna, onion, and mayonnaise. Spoon the mixture over two bread slices, top with mozzarella cheese, and cover with the remaining bread slices.

2. Brush with olive oil and arrange the sandwiches in the air fryer basket. Bake at 360 F for 6-8 minutes, turning once halfway through. Serve and enjoy!

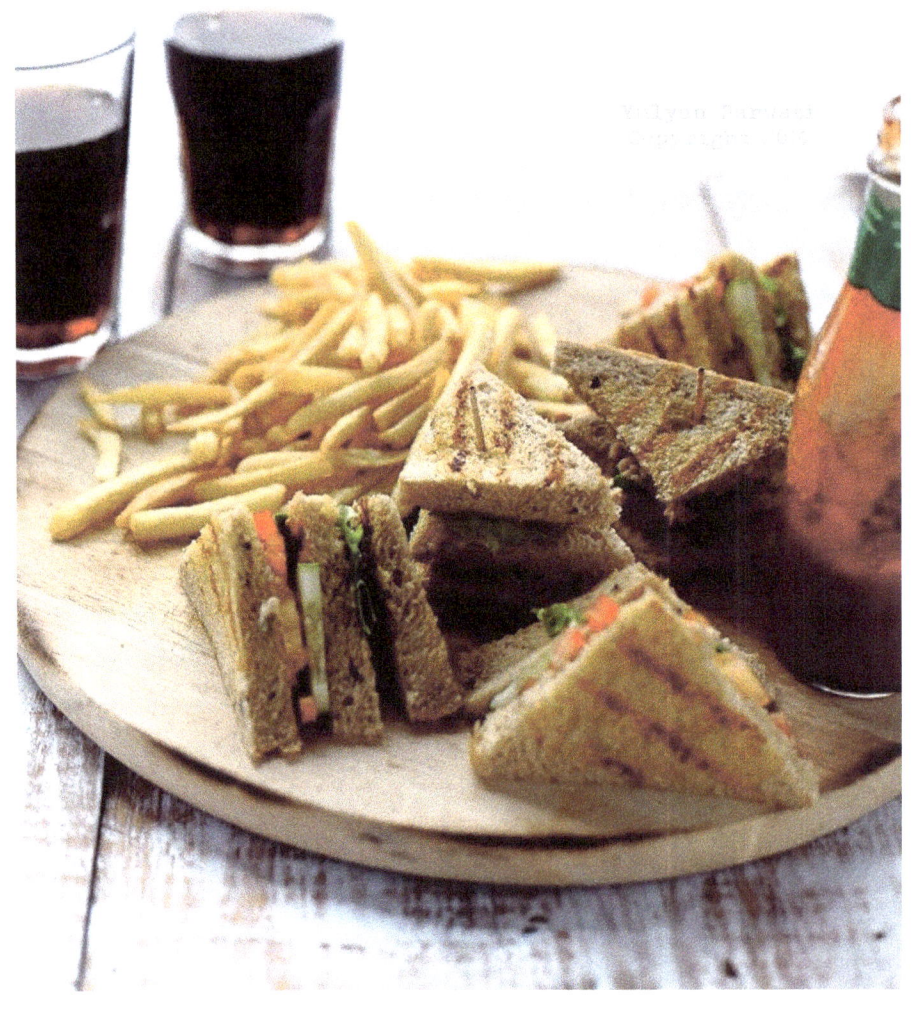

Greek-Style Fried Mussels

Cooking Time:

30 minutes

Servings: 4

Ingredients:

4 lb mussels

4 tbsp olive oil

1 cup white wine

Salt and black pepper to taste

1 tsp Greek seasoning

2 tbsp white wine vinegar

5 garlic cloves

4 bread slices

½ cup mixed nuts

Directions:

1. Preheat air fryer to 350 F. Add olive oil, garlic, Greek seasoning, vinegar, salt, mixed nuts, black pepper, and bread slices to a food processor and process until you obtain a creamy texture. In a skillet over medium heat, add wine and mussels.

2. Bring to a boil, then lower the heat and simmer until the mussels have opened up. Then, drain and remove from the shells.

3. Add them to the previously prepared mixture and toss to coat. Place in a greased baking dish and Bake in the air fryer for 10 minutes, shaking once. Serve warm.

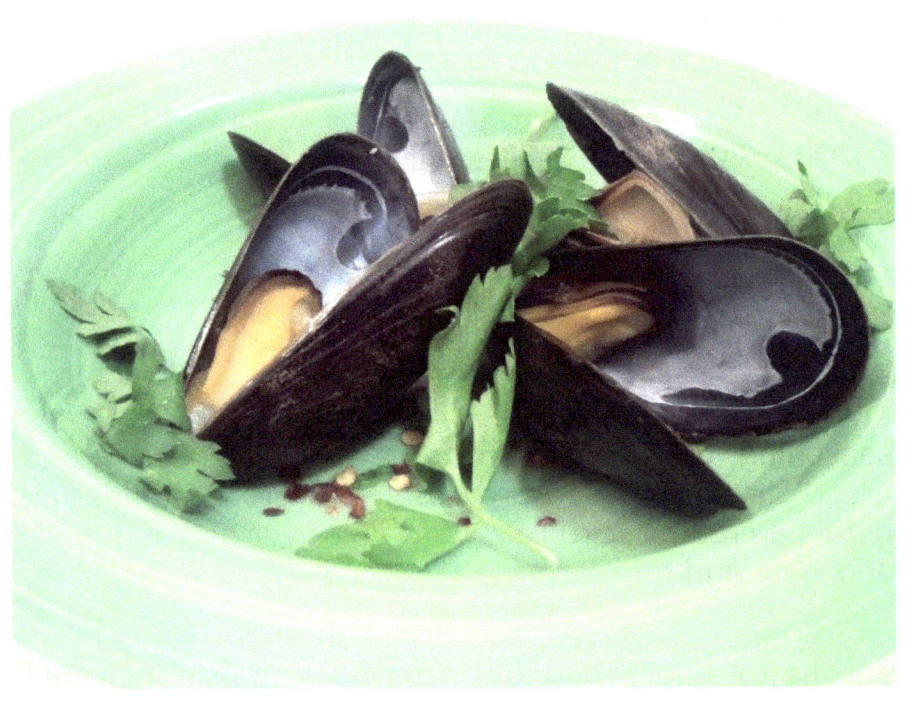

Greek-Style Salmon with Dill Sauce

Cooking Time:

20 minutes

Servings: 4

Ingredients:

1 lb salmon fillets

Salt and black pepper to taste

2 tsp olive oil

2 tbsp fresh dill, chopped

1 cup sour cream

1 cup Greek yogurt

Directions:

1.In a bowl, mix sour cream, yogurt, dill, and salt; set aside.

2.Preheat air fryer to 340 F. Drizzle olive oil over the salmon and rub with salt and black pepper. Arrange the fish in the frying basket and Bake for 10 minutes, flipping once. Top with the yogurt sauce .

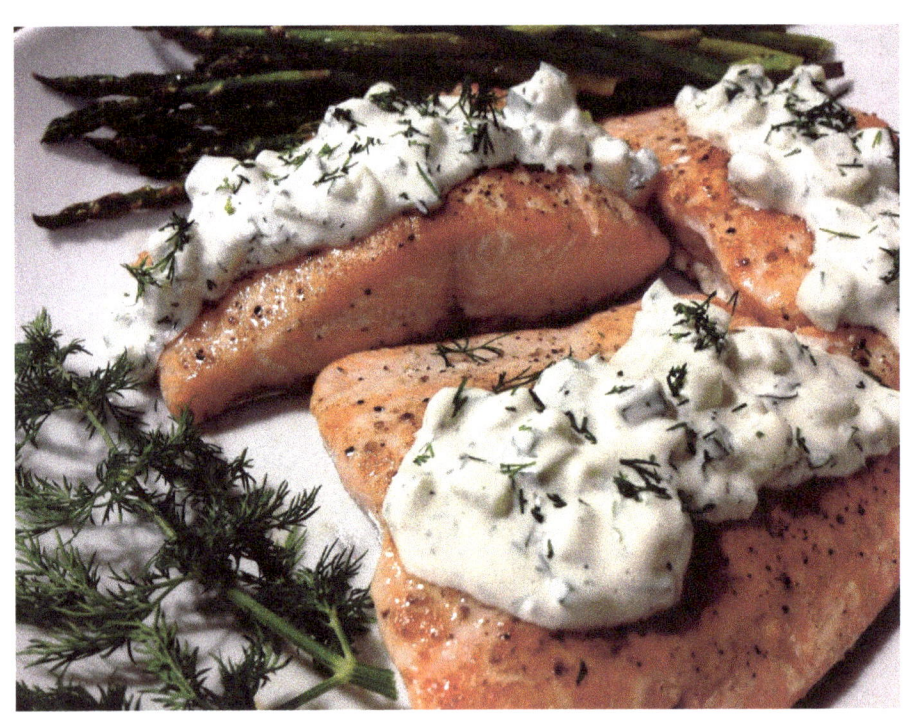

Simple Creole Trout

Cooking Time:

15 minutes

Servings: 4

Ingredients:

4 skin-on trout fillets

2 tsp creole seasoning

2 tbsp fresh dill, chopped

1 lemon, sliced

Directions:

1. Preheat air fryer to 350 F. Season the trout with creole seasoning on both sides and spray with cooking spray.

3. Place in the frying basket and Bake for 10-12 minutes, flipping once. Serve sprinkled with dill and garnished with lemon slices. Enjoy!

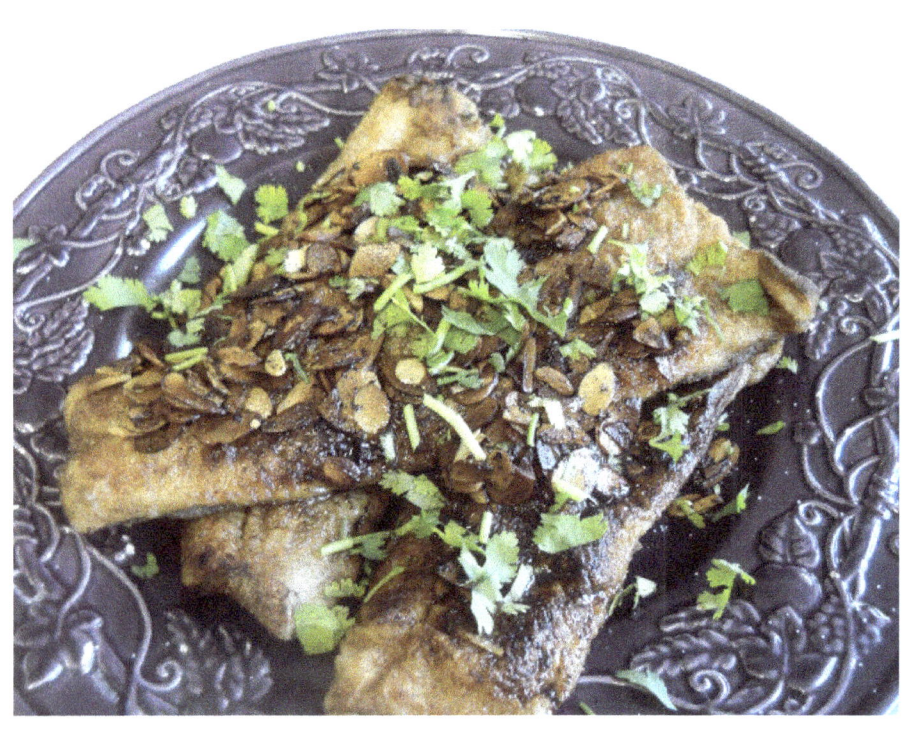

Colorful Salmon and Fennel Salad

Cooking Time:
20minutes
Servings:3
Ingredients:
1 pound salmon
1 fennel, quartered
1 teaspoon olive oil
Sea salt and ground black pepper, to taste
1/2 teaspoon paprika
1tablespoonbalsamicvinegar
1 tablespoon lime juice
1 tablespoon extra-virgin olive oil
1 tomato, sliced
1 cucumber, sliced
1 tablespoon sesame seeds, lightly toasted

Directions:

1.Toss the salmon and fennel with 1 teaspoon of olive oil, salt, black pepper and paprika.

2.Cook in the preheated Air Fryer at 380 degrees F for 12 minutes; shaking the basket once or twice. Cut the salmon into bite-sized strips and transfer them to a nice salad bowl.

3.Add in the fennel, balsamic vinegar, lime juice, 1 tablespoon of extra-virgin olive oil, tomato and cucumber. Toss to combine well and serve garnished with lightly toasted sesame seeds. Enjoy!

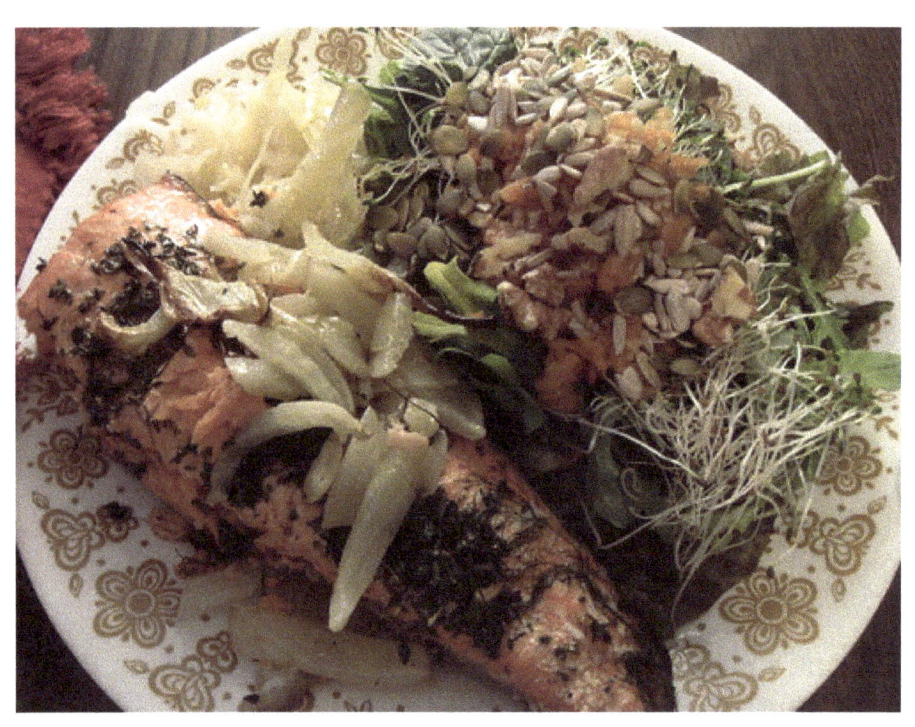

Fish Sticks with Vidalia Onions

Cooking Time:

12 minutes

Servings: 3

Ingredients:

1/2 pound fish sticks, frozen

1/2 pound Vidalia onions, halved

1 teaspoon sesame oil

Sea salt and ground black pepper, to taste

1/2 teaspoon red pepper flakes

4 tablespoons mayonnaise

4 tablespoons Greek-style yogurt

1/4 teaspoon mustard seeds

1 teaspoon chipotle chili in adobo, minced

Directions:

1. Drizzle the fish sticks and Vidalia onions with sesame oil.

2. Toss them with salt, black pepper and red pepper flakes. Transfer them to the Air Fryer cooking basket.

3. Cook the fish sticks and onions at 400 degreed F for 5 minutes. Shake the basket and cook an additional 5 minutes or until cooked through.

4. Meanwhile, mix the mayonnaise, Greek-style yogurt, mustard seeds and chipotle chili. Serve the warm fish sticks garnished with Vidalia onions and the sauce on the side. Serve and enjoy!

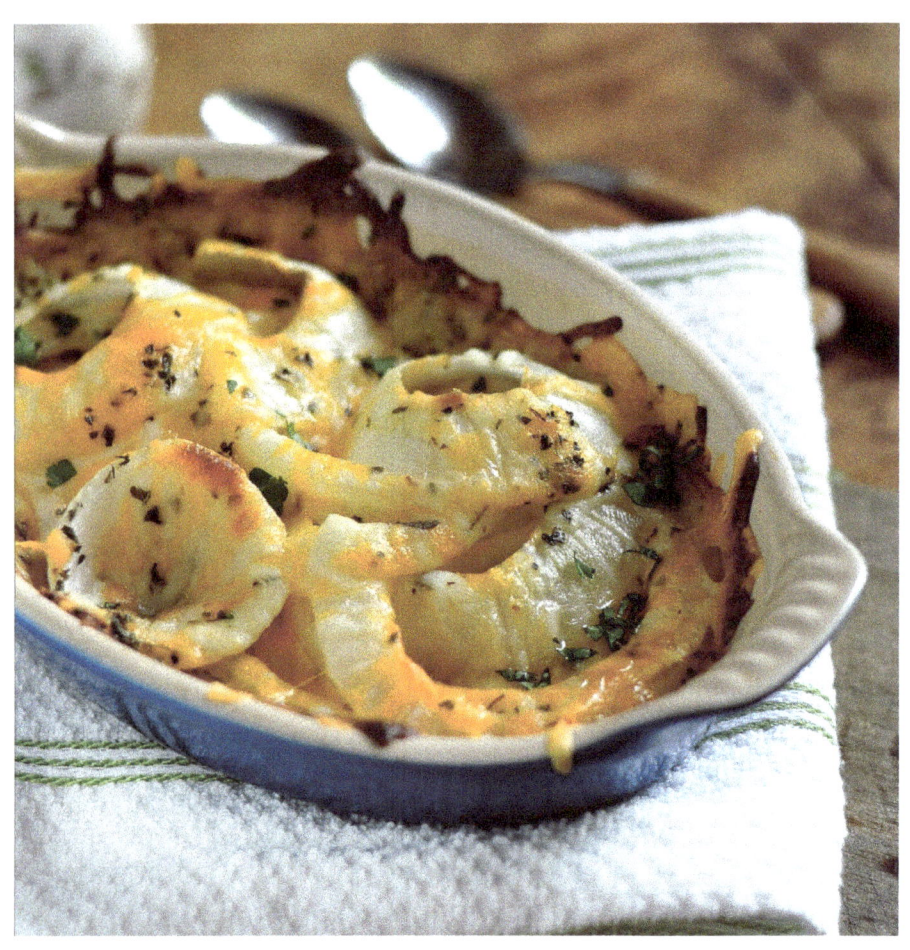

Fish Cakes with Bell Pepper

Cooking Tome:

15minutes

Servings:4

Ingredients:

1pound haddock

1 egg

2 tablespoons milk

1 bell pepper, deveined and finely chopped

2 stalks fresh scallions, minced

1/2 teaspoon fresh garlic, minced

Sea salt and ground black pepper, to taste

1/2 teaspoon cumin seeds

1/4 teaspoon celery seeds

1/2 cup breadcrumbs

1 teaspoon olive oil

Directions:

1.Thoroughly combine all ingredients, except for the breadcrumbs and olive oil, until everything is blended well.

2.Then, roll the mixture into 3 patties and coat them with breadcrumbs, pressing to adhere.

3.Drizzle olive oil over the patties and transfer them to the Air Fryer cooking basket.

4.Cook the fish cakes at 400 degrees F for 5 minutes; turn them over and continue to cook an additional 5 minutes until cooked through. Serve and enjoy!

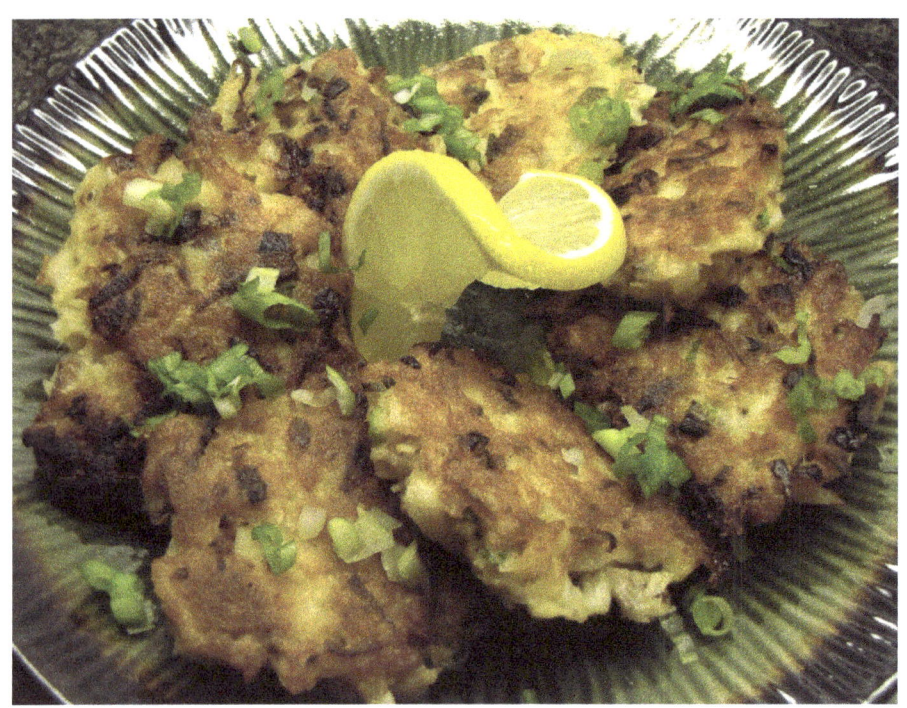

Cajun Fish Cakes with Cheese

Cooking Time:

30 minutes

Servings: 4

Ingredients:

1 catfish fillets

1 cup all-purpose flour

3 ounces butter

1 teaspoon baking powder

1 teaspoon baking soda

1/2 cup buttermilk

1 teaspoon Cajun seasoning

1 cup Swiss cheese, shredded

Directions:

1. Bring a pot of salted water to a boil. Boil the fish fillets for 5 minutes or until it is opaque. Flake the fish into small pieces.

2. Mix the remaining ingredients in a bowl; add the fish and mix until well combined. Shape the fish mixture into 12 patties.

3. Cook in the preheated Air Fryer at 380 degrees F for 15 minutes. Work in batches. Enjoy!

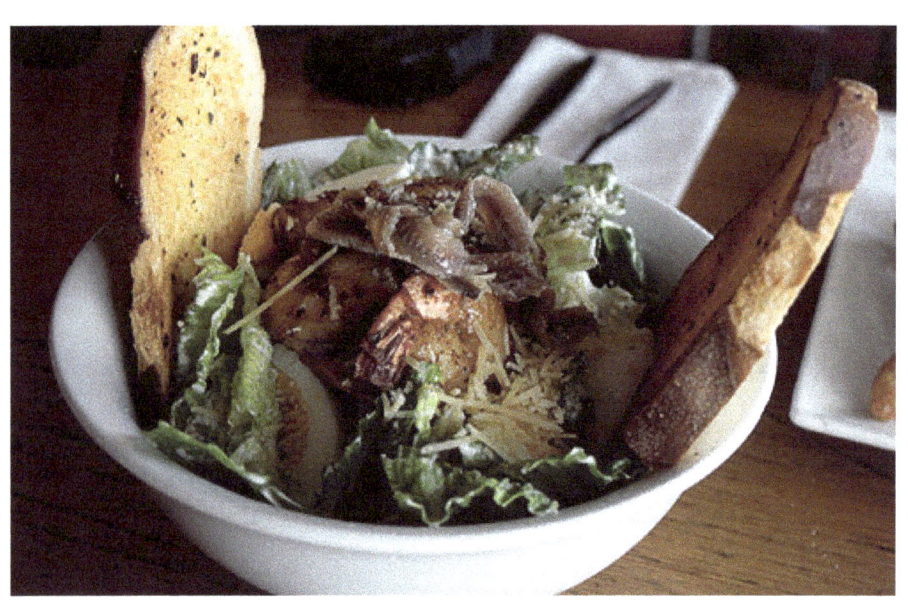

Monkfish with Sautéed Vegetables and Olives

Cooking Time:

20 minutes

Servings: 4

Ingrediengts:

2 teaspoons olive oil

2 carrots, sliced

2 bell peppers, sliced

1 teaspoon dried thyme

1/2 teaspoon dried marjoram

1/2 teaspoon dried rosemary

2 monkfish fillets

1 tablespoon soy sauce

2 tablespoons lime juice

Coarse Salt and ground black pepper, to taste

1 teaspoon cayenne pepper

1/2 cup Kalamata olives, pitted and sliced

Directions:

1. In a nonstick skillet, heat the olive oil for 1 minute. Once hot, sauté the carrots and peppers until tender, about 4 minutes.

2. Sprinkle with thyme, marjoram, and rosemary and set aside. Toss the fish fillets with the soy sauce, lime juice, salt, black pepper, and cayenne pepper.

3. Place the fish fillets in a lightly greased cooking basket and bake at 390 degrees F for 8 minutes.

4.Turn them over, add the olives, and cook an additional 4 minutes. Serve with the sautéed vegetables on the side. Enjoy!

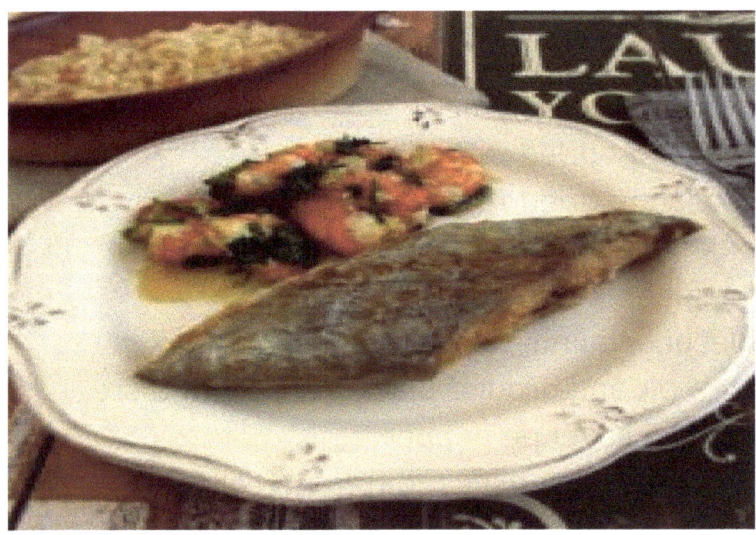

Crispy Mustardy Fish Fingers

Cooking Time:
20 minutes
Servings: 4
Ingredients:
1 ½ pounds tilapia pieces fingers
1/2 cup all-purpose flour
2 eggs
1 tablespoon yellow mustard
1 cup cornmeal
1 teaspoon garlic powder
1 teaspoon onion powder
Sea salt and ground black pepper, to taste
1/2 teaspoon celery powder
2 tablespoons peanut oil

Directions:

1. Pat dry the fish fingers with a kitchen towel. To make a breading station, place the all-purpose flour in a shallow dish.

2. In a separate dish, whisk the eggs with mustard. In a third bowl, mix the remaining ingredients.

3. Dredge the fish fingers in the flour, shaking the excess into the bowl; dip in the egg mixture and turn to coat evenly; then, dredge in the cornmeal mixture, turning a couple of times to coat evenly.

4.Cook in the preheated Air Fryer at 390 degrees F for 5 minutes; turn them over and cook another 5 minutes. Enjoy!

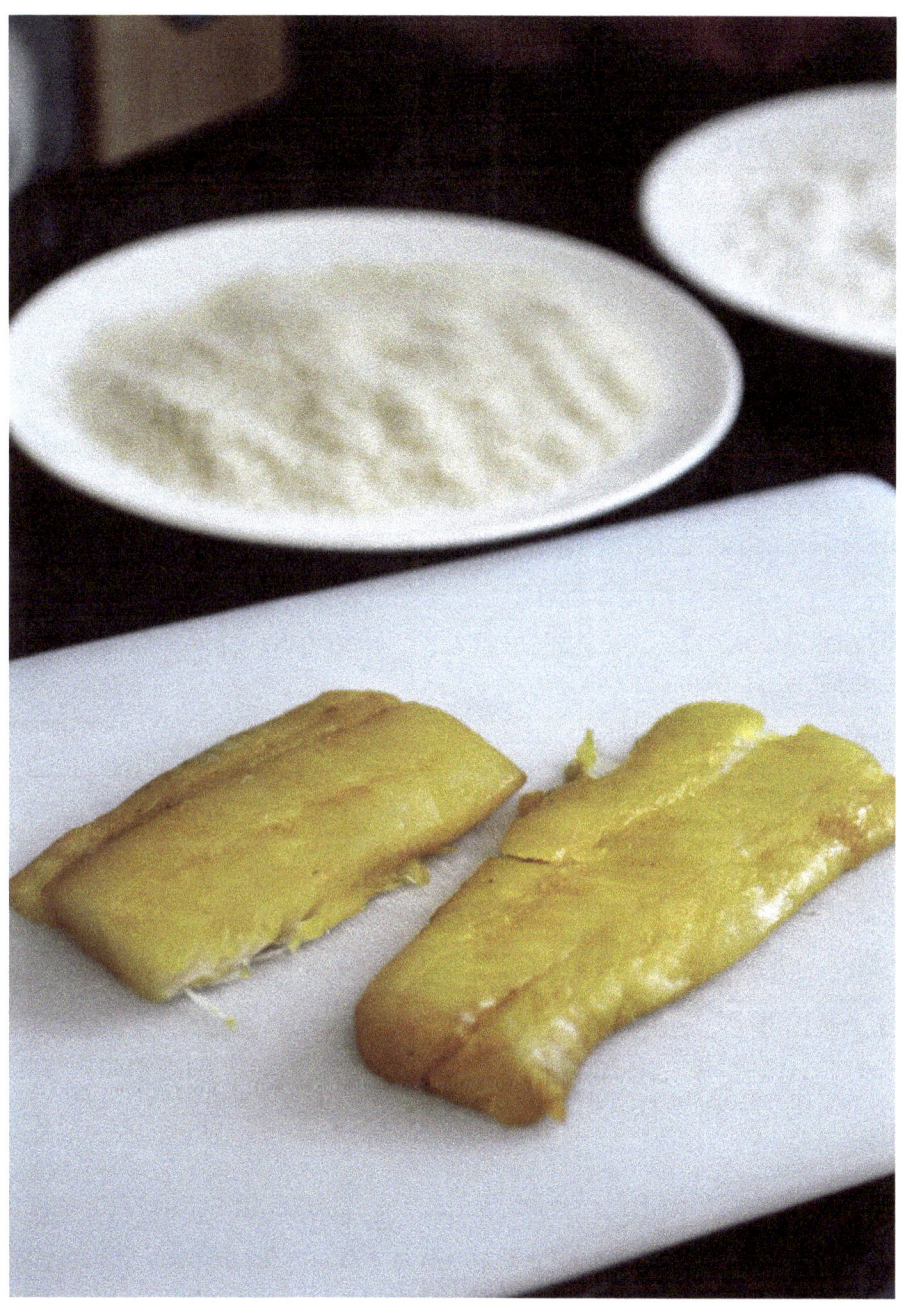

Roasted Mediterranean Snapper Fillets

Cook Time:

20 minutes

Servings: 3

Ingredients:

Marinade:

1 tablespoon black olives, chopped

1/4 cup dry white wine

2 tablespoons fresh lemon juice

1/2 teaspoon dried oregano

1/2 teaspoon dried basil

1 tablespoon parsley leaves, chopped

1 tomato, pureed

Roasted Snapper:

1 pound snapper fillets

1/2 cup cassava flour

Salt and white pepper, to taste

Directions:

1. Add all ingredients for the marinade to a large ceramic bowl. Add the snapper fillets and let them marinate for 1 hour in your refrigerator.

2. Place the cassava flour on a tray; now, coat the snapper fillets with the cassava flour. Season with salt and pepper.

3.Cook the snapper fillets in the preheated Air Fryer at 395 degrees F for 10 minutes, basting with the marinade and flipping them halfway through the cooking time. Serve and enjoy!

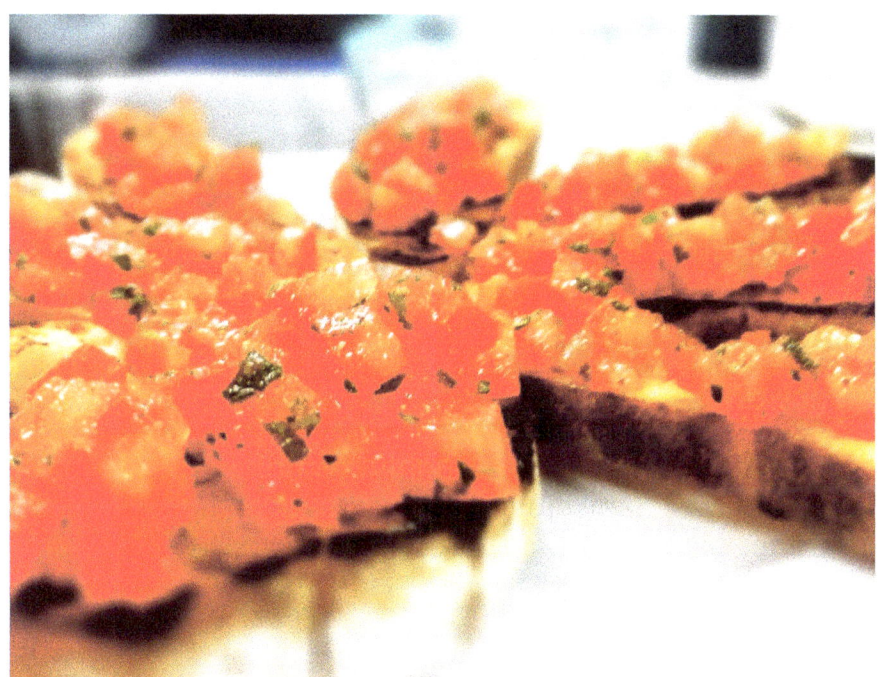

Quick Thai Coconut Fish

Cook Time:

20minutes

Servings: 4

Ingredients:

1 cup coconut milk
2 tablespoons lime juice
2 tablespoons Shoyu sauce
Salt and white pepper, to taste
1 teaspoon turmeric powder
1/2 teaspoon ginger powder
1/2 Thai Bird's Eye chili, seeded and finely chopped
1 pound tilapia
2 tablespoons olive oil

Directions:

1. In a mixing bowl, thoroughly combine the coconut milk with the lime juice, Shoyu sauce, salt, pepper, turmeric, ginger, and chili pepper.

2. Add tilapia and let it marinate for 1 hour. Brush the Air Fryer basket with olive oil.

3. Discard the marinade and place the tilapia fillets in the Air Fryer basket.

4. Cook the tilapia in the preheated Air Fryer at 400 degrees F for 6 minutes; turn them over and cook for 6 minutes more.

5.Work in batches. Serve with some extra lime wedges if desired. Enjoy!

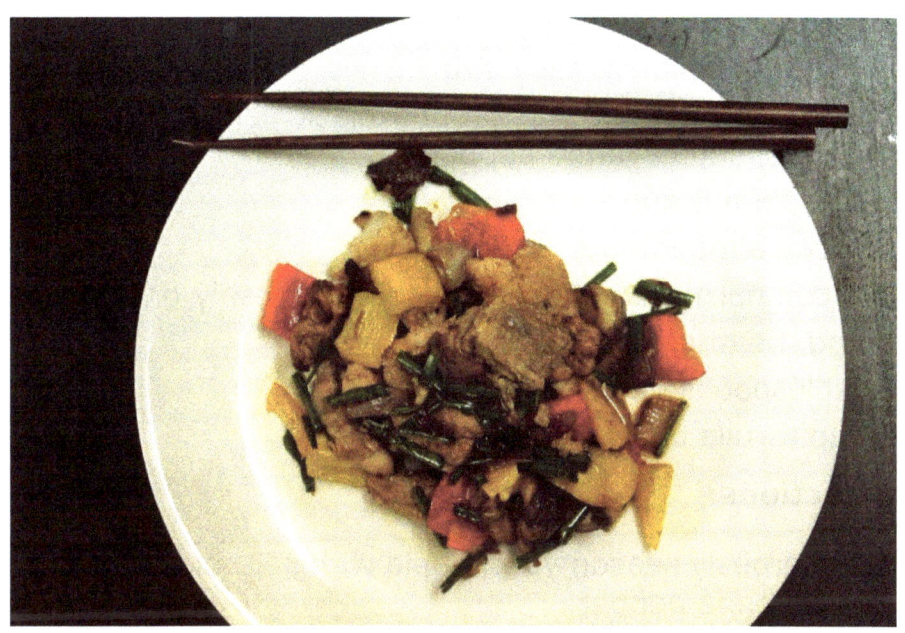

Parmesan Chip-Crusted Tilapia

Cooking Time:

15 minutes

Servings: 4

Ingredients:

1 ½ pounds tilapia, slice into

4 portions Sea salt and ground black pepper, to taste

1/2 teaspoon cayenne pepper

1 teaspoon granulated garlic

1/4 cup almond flour

1/4 cup parmesan cheese, preferably freshly grated

1 egg, beaten

2 tablespoons buttermilk

1 cup tortilla chips, crushed

Directions:

1. Generously season your tilapia with salt, black pepper and cayenne pepper.

2. Prepare a bread station. Add the granulated garlic, almond flour and parmesan cheese to a rimmed plate.

3. Whisk the egg and buttermilk in another bowl and place crushed tortilla chips in the third bowl.

4. Dip the tilapia pieces in the flour mixture, then in the egg/buttermilk mixture and finally roll them in the crushed chips, pressing to adhere well.

5.Cook in your Air Fryer at 400 degrees F for 10 minutes, flipping halfway through the cooking time. Serve with chips if desired. Enjoy!

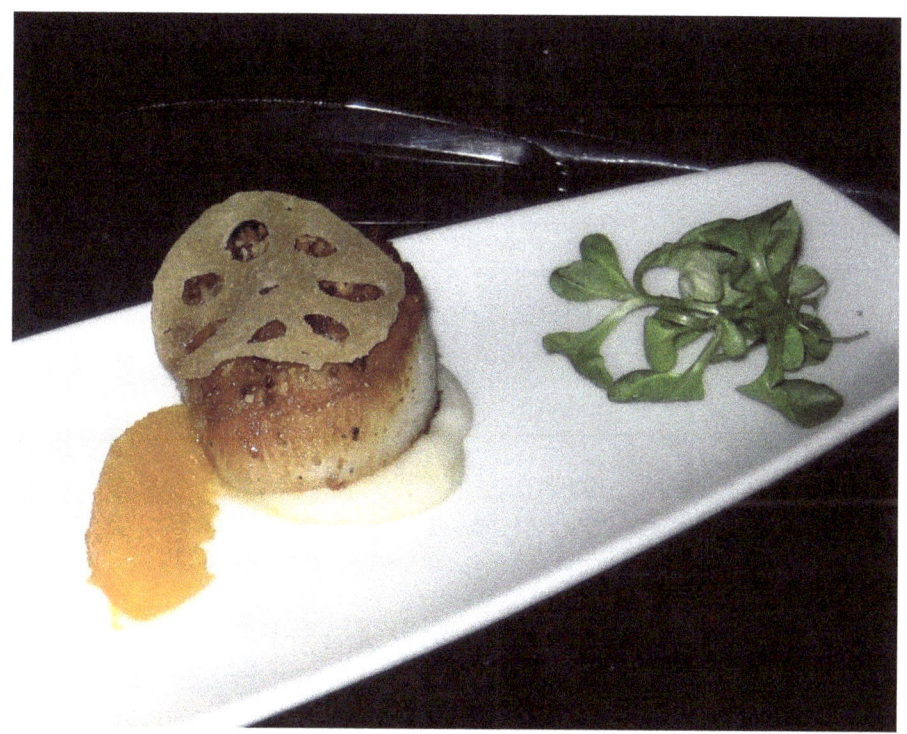

Classic Crab Cakes

Cooking Time:

15 minutes

Servings: 4

Ingredients:

1 egg, beaten

2 tablespoons milk

2 crustless bread slices

1 pound lump crabmeat

2 tablespoons scallions, chopped

1 garlic clove, minced

1 teaspoon deli mustard

1 teaspoon Sriracha sauce

Sea salt and ground black pepper, to taste

4 lemon wedges, for serving

Directions:

1. Whisk the egg and milk until pale and frothy; add in the bread and let it soak for a few minutes.

2. Stir in the other ingredients, except for the lemon wedges; shape the mixture into 4 equal patties.

3. Place your patties in the Air Fryer cooking basket. Spritz your patties with a nonstick cooking spray.

4. Cook the crab cakes at 400 degrees F for 5 minutes. Turn them over and cook on the other side for 5 minutes.

5.Serve warm, garnished with lemon wedges. Serve and enjoy!

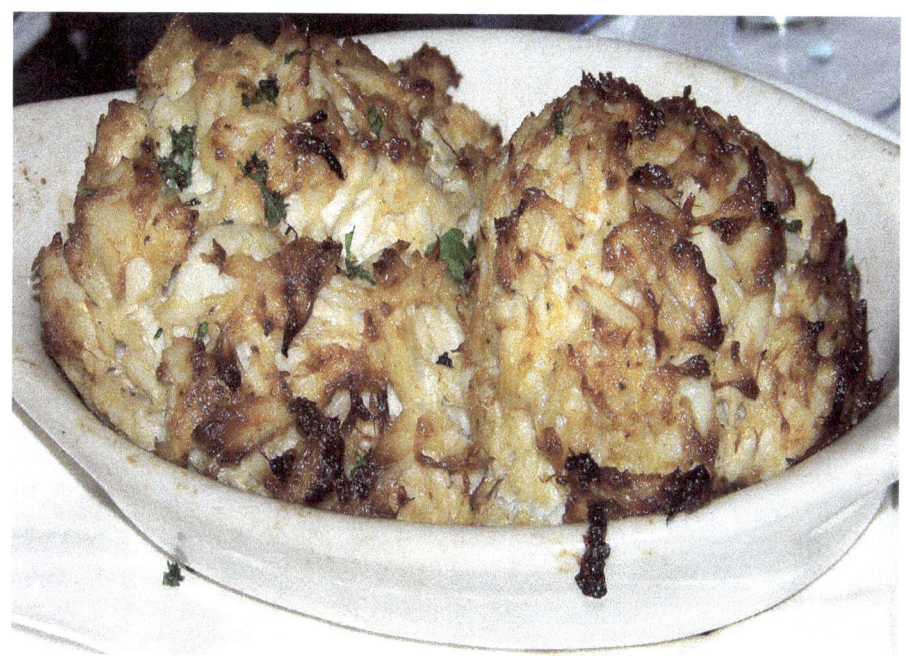

Baked Sardines with Tangy Dipping Sauce

Cooking Time:

45 minutes

Servings: 3

Ingredients:

1 pound fresh sardines

Sea salt and ground black pepper, to taste

1 teaspoon Italian seasoning mix

2 cloves garlic, minced

3 tablespoons olive oil

1/2 lemon, freshly squeezed

Directions:

1.Toss your sardines with salt, black pepper and Italian seasoning mix.

2.Cook in your Air Fryer at 325 degrees F for 35 to 40 minutes until skin is crispy.

3.Meanwhile, make the sauce by whisking the remaining ingredients Serve warm sardines with the sauce on the side. Serve and enjoy!

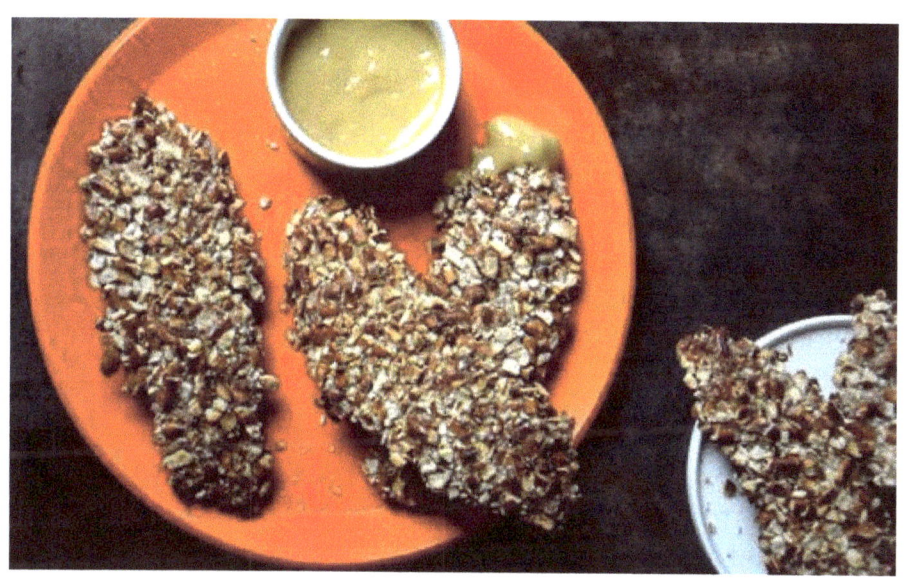

Classic Old Bay Fish with Cherry Tomatoes

Cooking Time:

15 minutes

Servings: 3

Ingredients:

1 pound swordfish steak

1/2 cup cornflakes, crushed

1 teaspoon Old Bay seasoning

Salt and black pepper, to season

2 teaspoon olive oil

1 pound cherry tomatoes

Directions:

1. Toss the swordfish steak with cornflakes, Old Bay seasoning, salt, black pepper and 1 teaspoon of olive oil.

2. Cook the swordfish steak in your Air Fryer at 400 degrees F for 6 minutes. Now, turn the fish over, top with tomatoes and drizzle with the remaining teaspoon of olive oil.

3. Continue to cook for 4 minutes. Serve with lemon slices if desired. Enjoy!

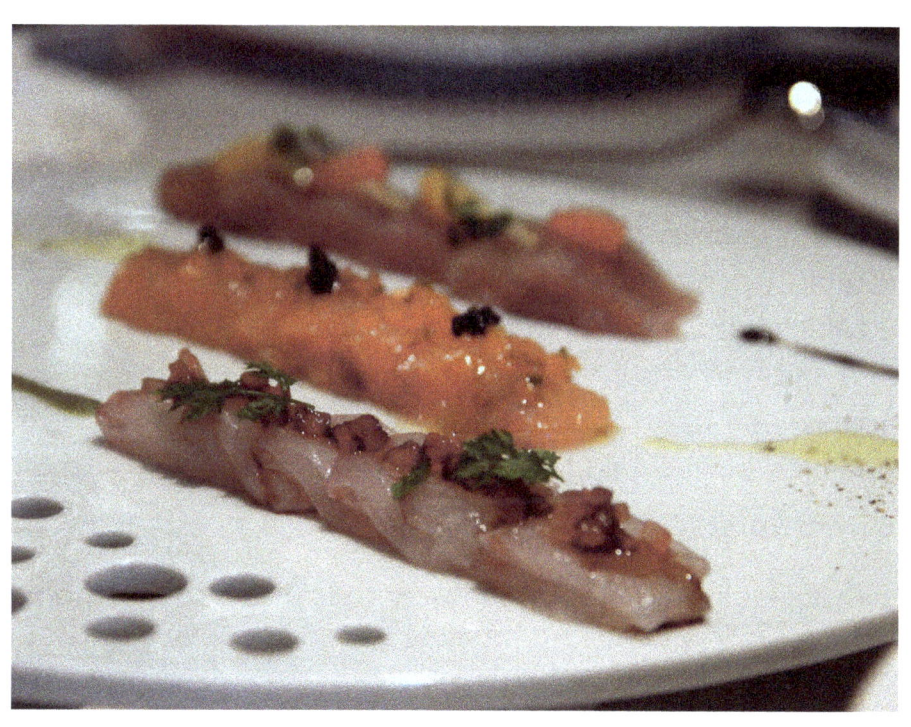

Mom's Lobster Tails

Cooking Time:

15 minutes

Servings: 4

Ingredients:

1/2 pound lobster tails

1 teaspoon olive oil

1 teaspoon fresh lime juice

1 bell pepper, sliced

1 jalapeno pepper, sliced

1 carrot, julienned

1 cup green cabbage, shredded

2 tablespoons mayonnaise

2 tablespoons Greek-style yogurt

Sea salt and ground black pepper, to taste

1 teaspoon baby capers, drained

4 leaves butterhead lettuce, for serving

Directions:

1. Drizzle olive oil over the lobster tails and transfer them to the Air Fryer cooking basket. Cook the lobster tails at 370 degrees F for 3 minutes.

2. Then, turn them over and cook on the other side for 3 to 4 minutes more until they are opaque.

3. Toss the lobster tails with the other ingredients, except for the lettuce leaves; gently stir until well combined.

4.Lay the lettuce leaves on a serving platter and top with the lobster salad. Enjoy!

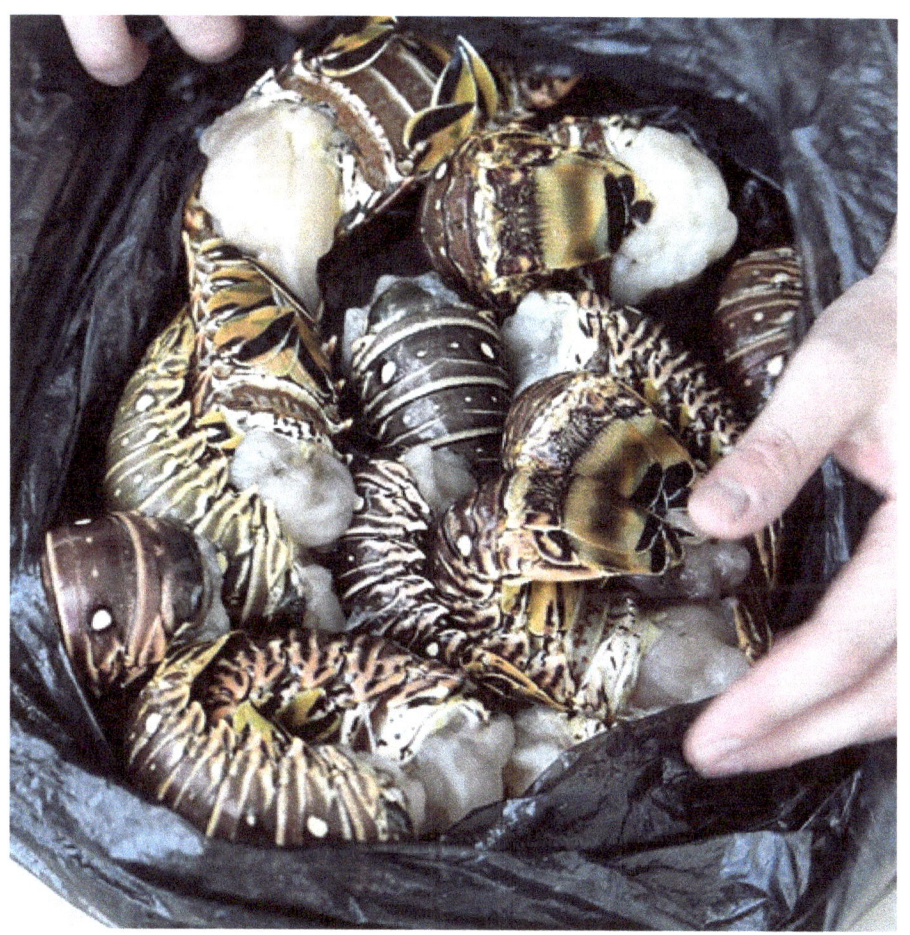

Tuna Steak with Roasted Cherry Tomatoes

Cooking Time:
30 minutes

Servings: 3

Ingredients:

1 pound tuna steak

1 cup cherry tomatoes

1 teaspoon extra-virgin olive oil

2 sprigs rosemary, leaves picked and crushed

Sea salt and red pepper flakes, to taste

1 teaspoon garlic, finely chopped

1 tablespoon lime juice

Directions:

1. Toss the tuna steaks and cherry tomatoes with olive oil, rosemary leaves, salt, black pepper and garlic.

2. Place the tuna steaks in a lightly oiled cooking basket; cook tuna steaks at 440 degrees F for about 6 minutes. Turn the tuna steaks over, add in the cherry tomatoes and continue to cook for 4 minutes more.

3. Drizzle the fish with lime juice and serve warm garnished with roasted cherry tomatoes! Enjoy!

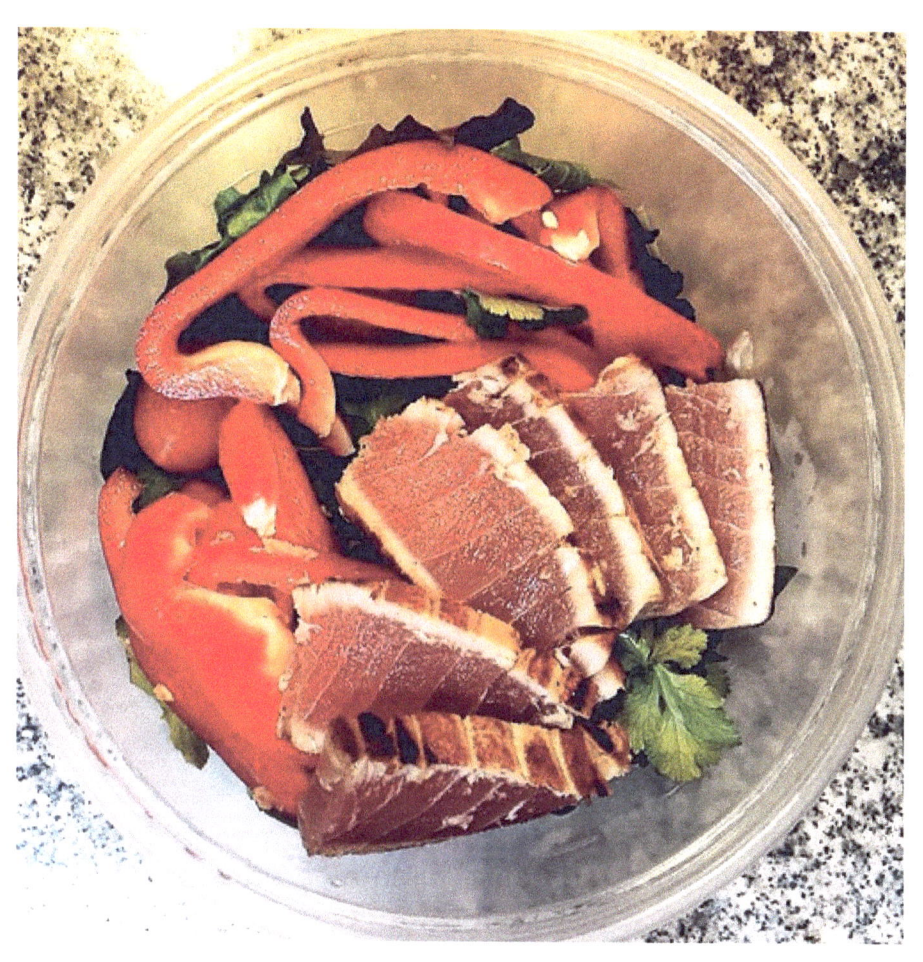

Vermouth and Garlic Shrimp Skewers

Cook Time:

15minutes

Servings:4

INGREDIENTS

1½ pounds shrimp

1/4 cup vermouth

2 cloves garlic, crushed

1 teaspoon dry mango powder

Kosher salt, to taste

1/4 teaspoon black pepper, freshly ground

2 tablespoons olive oil

4 tablespoons flour

8 skewers, soaked in water for 30 minutes

1 lemon, cut into wedges

DIRECTIONS

1.Add the shrimp, vermouth, garlic, mango powder, salt, black pepper, and olive oil in a ceramic bowl; let it sit for 1 hour in your refrigerator.

2.Discard the marinade and toss the shrimp with flour. Thread on to skewers and transfer to the lightly greased cooking basket.

3.Cook at 400 degrees F for 5 minutes, tossing halfway through. Serve with lemon wedges. Enjoy!

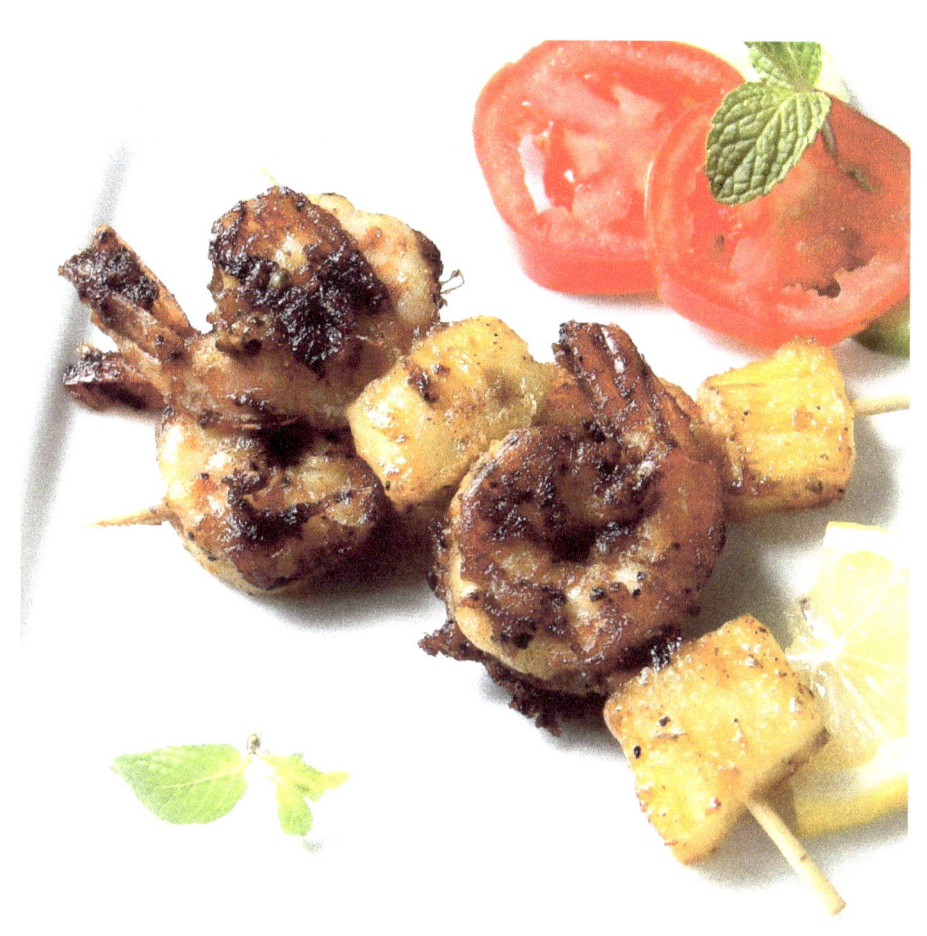

Cod and Shallot Frittata

Cooking Time:

30minutes

Servings:3

Ingredients:

1cod fillets

6 eggs

1/2 cup milk

1 shallot, chopped

2 garlic cloves, minced

Sea salt and ground black pepper, to taste

1/2 teaspoon red pepper flakes, crushed

DIRECTIONS

1.Bring a pot of salted water to a boil. Boil the cod fillets for 5 minutes or until it is opaque. Flake the fish into bite-sized pieces.

2.In a mixing bowl, whisk the eggs and milk. Stir in the shallots, garlic, salt, black pepper, and red pepper flakes.

3.Stir in the reserved fish. Pour the mixture into the lightly greased baking pan. Cook in the preheated Air Fryer at 360 degrees F for 9 minutes, flipping over halfway through.

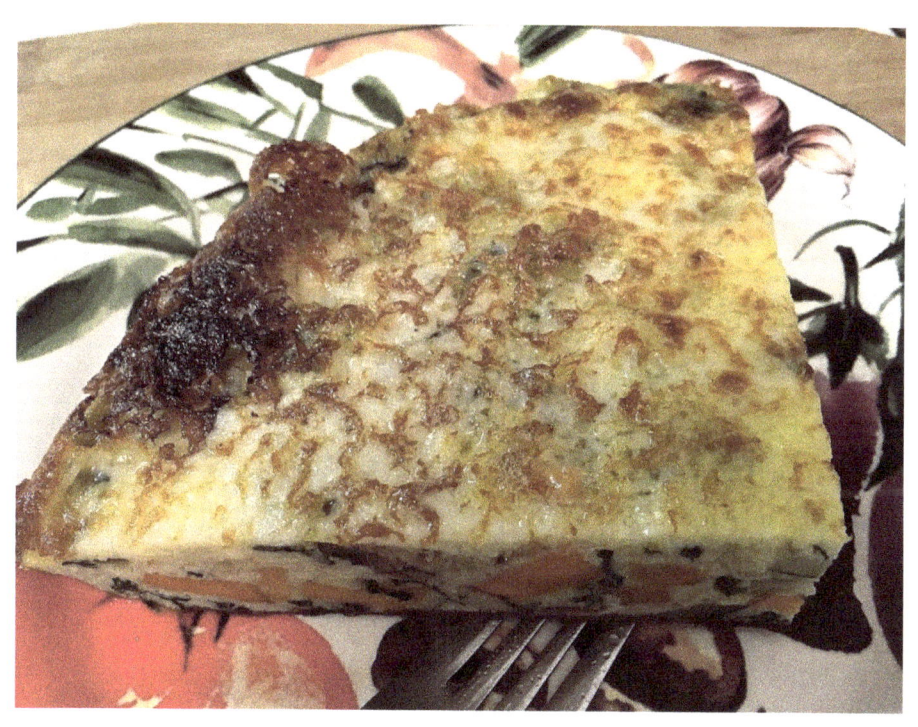

Authentic Mediterranean Calamari Salad

Cooking Time:
15 minutes
Servings: 3
Ingredients:
1 pound squid, cleaned, sliced into rings
2 tablespoons sherry wine
1/2 teaspoon granulated garlic
Salt, to taste
1/2 teaspoon ground black pepper
1/2 teaspoon basil
1/2 teaspoon dried rosemary
1 cup grape tomatoes
1 small red onion, thinly sliced
1/3 cup Kalamata olives, pitted and sliced
1/2 cup mayonnaise
1 teaspoon yellow mustard
1/2 cup fresh flat-leaf parsley leaves, coarsely chopped

Directions:

1. Start by preheating the Air Fryer to 400 degrees F. Spritz the Air Fryer basket with cooking oil.

2. Toss the squid rings with the sherry wine, garlic, salt, pepper, basil, and rosemary.

3. Cook in the preheated Air Fryer for 5 minutes, shaking the basket halfway through the cooking time. Work in batches and let it cool to room temperature.

3.When the squid is cool enough, add the remaining ingredients. Gently stir to combine and serve well chilled. Enjoy!

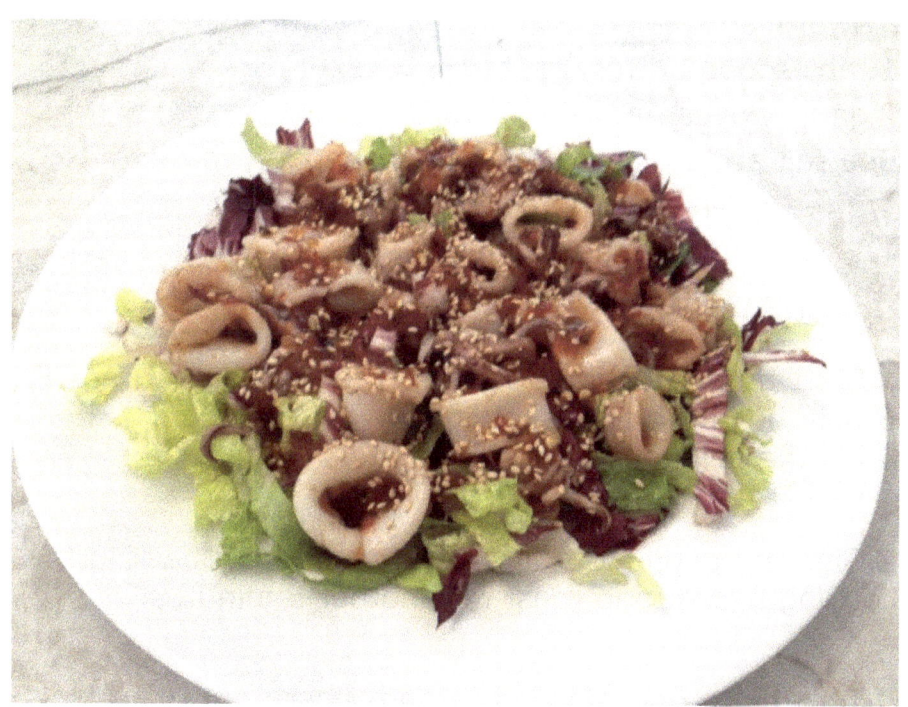

Swordfish with Roasted Peppers and Garlic Sauce

Cooking Time:
30 minutes
Servings: 4
Ingredients:
3 bell peppers
3 swordfish steaks
1 tablespoon butter, melted
2 garlic cloves, minced
Sea salt and freshly ground black pepper, to taste
1/2 teaspoon cayenne pepper
1/2 teaspoon ginger powder

Directions:

1. Start by preheating your Air Fryer to 400 degrees F. Brush the Air Fryer basket lightly with cooking oil. Then, roast the bell peppers for 5 minutes.

2. Give the peppers a half turn; place them back in the cooking basket and roast for another 5 minutes.

3. Turn them one more time and roast until the skin is charred and soft or 5 more minutes. Peel the peppers and set aside.

4. Then, add the swordfish steaks to the lightly greased cooking basket and cook at 400 degrees F for 10 minutes.

5.Meanwhile, melt the butter in a small saucepan. Cook the garlic until fragrant and add the salt, pepper, cayenne pepper, and ginger powder.

6.Cook until everything is thoroughly heated. Plate the peeled peppers and the roasted swordfish; spoon the sauce over them and serve warm. Enjoy!

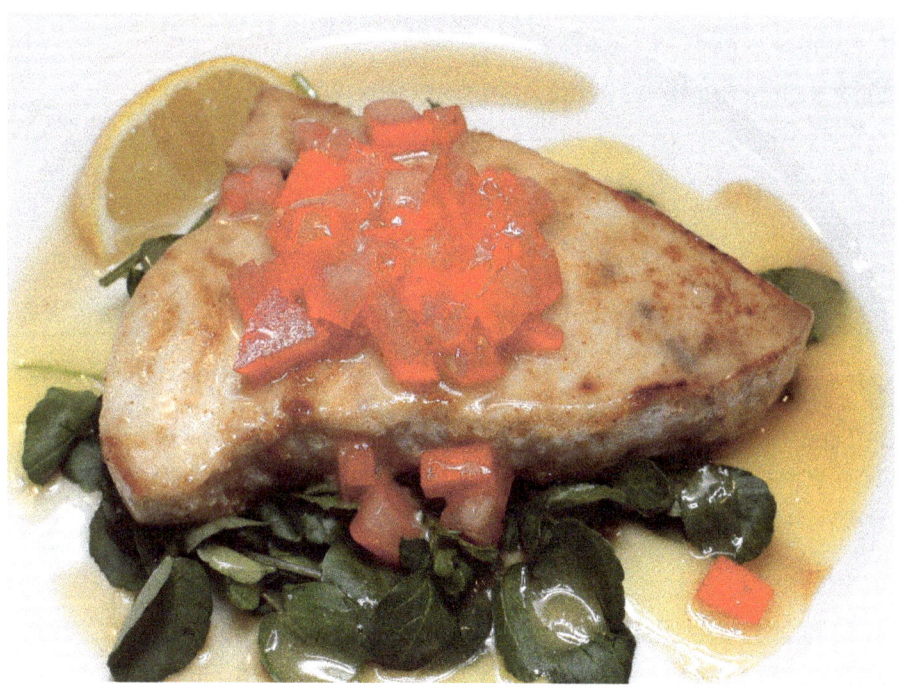

Shrimp Kabobs with Cherry Tomatoes

Cooking Time:
30minutes
Servings:4
Ingredients:
1½ pounds jumbo shrimp, cleaned, shelled and deveined
1 pound cherry tomatoes
2 tablespoons butter, melted
1 tablespoons Sriracha sauce
Sea salt and ground black pepper, to taste
1/2 teaspoon dried oregano
1/2 teaspoon dried basil
1 teaspoon dried parsley flakes
1/2 teaspoon marjoram
1/2 teaspoon mustard seeds

Directions:

1.Toss all ingredients in a mixing bowl until the shrimp and tomatoes are covered on all sides. Soak the wooden skewers in water for 15 minutes.

2.Thread the jumbo shrimp and cherry tomatoes onto skewers. Cook in the preheated Air Fryer at 400 degrees F for 5 minutes, working with batches.

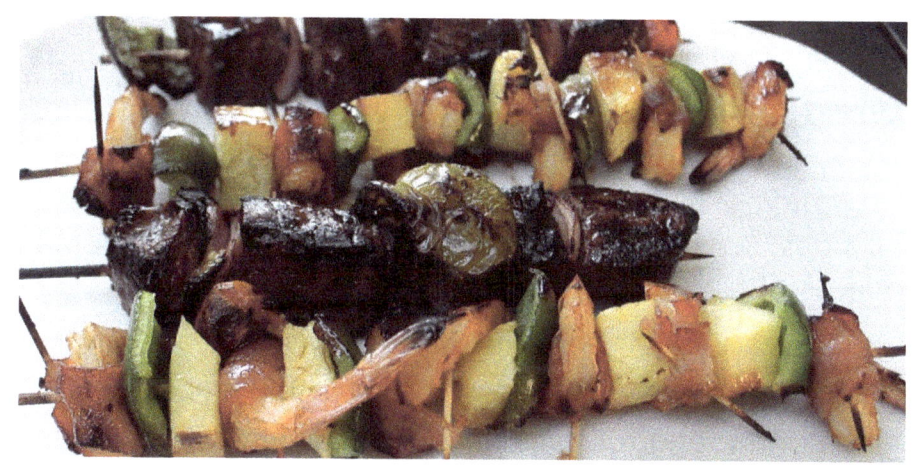

Keto Cod Fillets

Cooking Time:
15 minutes
Servings:4
Ingredients:
1cod fish fillets
1 teaspoon butter, melted
1 teaspoon Old Bay seasoning
1 egg, beaten
2 tablespoons coconut milk, unsweetened
1/3 cup coconut flour, unsweetened

Directions:

1.Place the cod fish fillets, butter and Old Bay seasoning in a Ziplock bag; shake until the fish is well coated on all sides. In a shallow bowl, whisk the egg and coconut milk until frothy.

2.In another bowl, place the coconut flour. Dip the fish fillets in the egg mixture, then, coat them with coconut flour, pressing to adhere.

3.Cook the fish at 390 degrees F for 6 minutes; flip them over and cook an additional 6 minutes until your fish flakes easily when tested with a fork. Serve and enjoy!

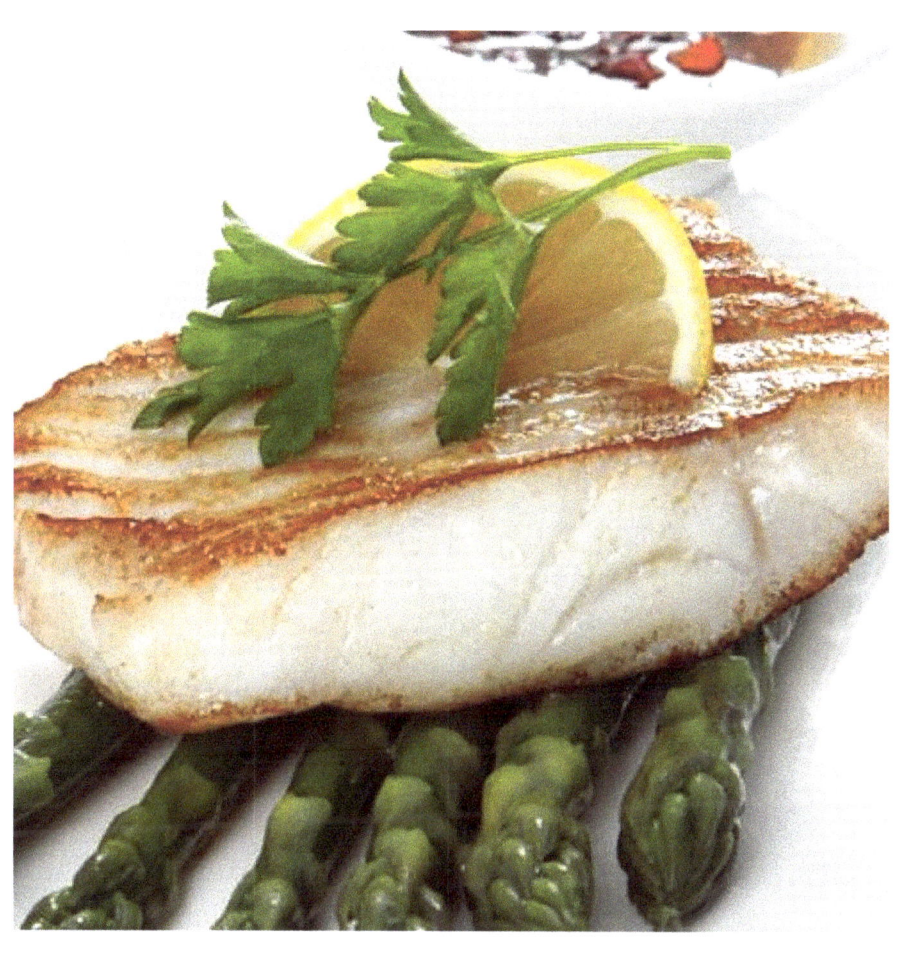

www.ingramcontent.com/pod-product-compliance
Lightning Source LLC
Chambersburg PA
CBHW071108030426
42336CB00013BA/2005